# As Lovers Do

GOD SAID TO ADAM AND EVE, "I HAVE TWO GIFTS, ONE FOR EACH."

SPYING THE RUBBERY THING IN GOD'S RIGHT HAND, ADAM ASKED, "LORD WHAT THAT?"

AND GOD REPLIED, "IT IS A PENIS. WITH IT YOU WOULD BE ABLE TO HAVE SEX A PISS STANDING UP."

AND ADAM SAID, "OH, THAT IS FOR ME," AS HE RAN OUTSIDE TO PEE HIS NAME THE SAND AND OTHERWISE PLAY WITH HIS NEW TOY.

GOD TURNED TO EVE AND HELD UP THE GREY LUMP IN HIS LEFT HAND, SAYING, "MY WORD, I DO NOT UNDERSTAND HUMAN FREE WILL. I WAS CERTAIN HE WOU WANT THIS BRAIN. AH WELL, I WILL GIVE IT TO YOU."

# As Lovers Do

## SEXUAL AND ROMANTIC PARTNERSHIP AS A PATH OF TRANSFORMATION

Marc Beneteau

Tranquility Consulting LLC
Philadelphia

**As Lovers Do**

ISBN
978-1515211631

Tranquility Consulting LLC
Philadelphia, PA
*www.AsLoversDo.com*

# Table of Contents

How to Use this Book.................................................................................8

Abstract....................................................................................................9


## PART 1: INTRODUCTION..............................................................12

1 Who this Book Is for?.......................................................................13

2 The Problem of Sexual Loving, Part 1.............................................20

3 The Nature of Personal Power.........................................................25

4 The War Between the Sexes.............................................................27

5 The Problem of Sexual Loving, Part 2.............................................31

6 Supporting Women vs. Being a Servant..........................................37


## PART 2: FOUNDATIONS.................................................................40

7 We Live in a Culture of Lying [Dieter Duhm] ...............................41

8 Skills and Principles of Loving [Jerry Jud].....................................45

9 Sexual Polarity [David Deida, Victor Baranco] ..............................54


## PART 3: BASIC MAN/WOMAN........................................................60

10 Seduction 101: Women Call, Men Respond [Victor Baranco] ......61

11 Self-Investment and the Paradox of Female Sexual Attraction [Mark Manson] ...............................................................................................65

12 Understanding and Executing the Feminine Commands..............74

13 The Importance of Authenticity.....................................................82

14 Responding to Negative Feedback from a Woman.........................84

15 What You Should Never Say to a Woman.......................................89

16 Initiating and Maintaining a Conversation....................................90

17 Complimenting and Flirting...........................................................95

18 Escalation: You Have Rapport. Or Not..........................................97

19 The Fundamental Problem of Women.............................................99

**PART 4: ADVANCED MAN/WOMAN**.......................................**104**

20 Feminism and the Rise of "Whole and Complete"............................... 105

21 Masculine Terms............................................................................... 112

22 What To Do When You Really Want to "Make Her Wrong"............... 120

23 Dealing With Feminine Resistance: the Dark Feminine, and the Deep
Feminine .......................................................................................... 122

24 Delving deeper into Masculine Purpose............................................ 130

25 Educating Yourself, Teaching Her to Ask for What She Wants, and
Avoiding Pitfalls............................................................................... 134

26 Handling Disinterest or Lack of Attraction....................................... 137

27 How to End a Relationship ............................................................... 141

**PART 5: SEXUALITY** ......................................................**144**

28 Human Sexuality 101: the Sea of Misinformation............................ 145

29 Women's "Over-Pleasing" ................................................................ 149

30 The Do-Date Technique of Clitoral Massage [Victor Baranco]........ 152

31 Sexual Variations, Games, and Fetishes .......................................... 161

32 Negotiating Sexual Differences: Sexual Chemistry and Problems of Desire
163

33 Sacred Sexuality and the Stages of Relationship [Chris Menné].......... 164

**PART 6: THE MAN/WOMAN GAME IN CULTURE AND PHILOSOPHY .
174**

34 The Inner Game of Masculine and Feminine [Shirley Luthman] ........... 175

35 Spiritual Underpinnings of Sexual Polarity, and the Future of Love....... 182

**PART 7: COMMUNICATION TOOLS AND RESOURCES** ....................**186**

36 Non-Violent Communication ........................................................... 187

37 Withholds ........................................................................................ 189

38 Hexes................................................................................................ 198

39 Anti-negotiations [Alison Armstrong]............................................. 199

40 You don't need to get what you want if you can express what you want200

41 Training Organizations ............................................................... 202

42 Bibliography .................................................................................. 206

Acknowledgements............................................................................ 209

# How to Use this Book

This book is not a mere philosophy of love and sex. It is an actionable manual, and as such, you will need to do the work. Here is my suggestion for preparing your practice.

Start by reading the **Abstract** and **Chapter 1**. If it resonates, keep on reading as that will give you the conceptual framework of the work and the more subtle distinctions, before you actually engage the practice.

But if the first few chapters don't resonate, or the ideas seem too abstract, don't give up. Skip forward and read **Chapter 12: Executing the Feminine Commands** and **Chapter 14: Responding to Negative Feedback**. These two chapters describe the fundamental action steps of masculine love: we attempt to love (serve or contribute to others), then we get feedback on how well we are doing, and lastly adjust. If you do nothing but that, you will have spectacular relationships.

This book is written from a masculine viewpoint. If you think you might be primarily feminine, follow the same process as for masculine people, for two reasons. First, you will be functioning in a masculine mode for large parts of your life, such as at your job and with your children, so the skills you will learn here will serve you. Second, it will give you empathy for the masculine experience, which will make you more lovable (attractive). In a later edition of the book, I hope to expand on the practice of feminine love. For now, you will need to read between the lines, or use the cited authors work, especially David Deida and Alison Armstrong.

Good luck!

# Abstract

*"Sexuality is the #1 super-power" – Dieter Duhm*

As Lovers Do is a practical guide for building community, increasing the number and quality of your intimate relationships, and having better sex. It is an integration of the work of many beloved and powerful teachers. Some of these teachers are still with us, others have passed-on; some are well known and others not; but all of them built significant learning communities. The integration of these teachings results in an intellectually compelling, practical and useful system for creating intentional loving community and for helping men and women get along better.

*"Love"* is defined as the act of giving other people what they want and need for their own happiness and growth [Scott Peck and Jerry Jud]. We do this is by increasing the quality of our attention, communication and appreciation [Dale Carnegie, Marshall Rosenberg, Werner Erhard]. ***The currency of love is attention and appreciation.***

A further distinction on love is provided by concepts of **Sexual Polarity** [David Deida, Victor Baranco, Alison Armstrong]. Masculine and Feminine are ways of being that we choose in the moment, and we may make a difference choice in the next moment. In our post-conventional, feminist society, we tend to ridicule and deny the reality of sexual polarity under the belief that human beings are androgynous. In many cases this equality creates a loss of happiness and power as we end up suppressing our real nature. ***We often imagine that our intimate partners can instinctively understand how we think and feel. They can't. We need to learn their language.***

On a personal level, this book is for men and women who want to have better relationships, both sexual and social. It is particularly effective for men seeking to attract women because it is compatible with a new seduction model called *"honest attraction"* [Mark Manson].

On a political level, it presents a plan for ending patriarchy and systemic violence in the world. This idea is inspired by Dieter Duhm's words: *"There can be no peace on earth as long as there is war in love,"* suggesting that healing relationships between men and women and finding fulfilling sexual expression is the most immediate and impactful thing we can do to put humanity back on the path of love. It's also a very fun game.

The path to true personal power in our complex world lies through deeper partnership and collaboration, which are other words for love. The outcome of this process is greater happiness and greater success or freedom — these being aspects of feminine and masculine goals, goals that support and complement each other perfectly, but whose simultaneous achievement has so far eluded most of us, and humanity as a whole as well.

*"Men and women have searched for each other for generations and always missed one another"* [Dieter Duhm]. This book is an attempt to explain why we have so much trouble connecting and what can be done about it. We have the capacity to transform our relationships with all the people in our lives, starting immediately with our intimate partners.

# PART 1: INTRODUCTION

The 30,000 foot overview: what you can expect from applying the lessons in this book, and a first pass on some important concepts and distinctions of human loving and sexual polarity.

# 1 Who this Book Is for?

*"Relationship is the quick path." – Chogyam Trungpa*

## Why read this book?

This is a book for men who want to relate more successfully and more powerfully to women. It is for men who want to live their lives as the fullest possible expression of their love and of their purpose, and who want their relationships with women to reflect that.

I am also writing for women who want to understand men better in order to bring out the best from them and relate to them more lovingly. Indeed, the type of shift advocated here can be initiated by either men or women, and their partners usually will respond. However, I am going to focus primarily on the masculine side of the Man/Woman game, simply because I am a man and therefore I cannot claim to fully understand women, and must be cautious in giving them advice... even, and especially, for their own good. Men's ideas on what is good for women are almost always off base.

You may be single and horny and looking for a way to attract women and then relate to them in a way that is authentic to you, and yet successful. You may already have one or more lovers, but find yourself struggling to understand them and what they want from you, what you yourself want, and what you actually have to give.

This book describes a way of life: men and women living inside an inter-dependent network of active communication, feedback, and appreciation – a network of love, a culture of acknowledgement and affirmation. This way of life can be hard work, and is not for everyone, but if the idea resonates, please read on.

Many of the attitudes and communication practices described here are universal, and will generate greater closeness and collaboration with anyone, man or woman. In fact, some of these ideas go back to commonsense but powerful relationship practices first articulated by Dale Carnegie, and later by Marshall Rosenberg's book **NON-VIOLENT**

**COMMUNICATION.** Even if you are not motivated by sexual intimacy at this point in your life, you might find these ideas useful.

In my own case, however, my life did not take off until I started applying these communication practices, and sexual polarity theory, to my relationships with women. It took me a very long time to figure all this out – two-thirds of a lifetime, more or less. I had some wise and powerful teachers, or I would never have learned at all. I hope you will not need to spend two-thirds of your life to just understand the basics, as I did. You will get it, and your life will take off.

This book is in a new class of relationship books that might be called **"honest attraction"** [Mark Manson]. Manson's idea that the key for men to attract women is to *invest in themselves,* and from there to become more discerning, authentic, and vulnerable men. Such men have higher quality attention on women because they have less attention on themselves. By investing in ourselves, we naturally move into a space of wanting to contribute to women. This is both more effective and more fun than traditional seduction techniques. We go deeply into Manson's ideas in Chapter 11.

> ### *DALE CARNEGIE (1888-1955)*
> *Dale Carnegie was a writer, speaker and the developer of famous courses in self-improvement, salesmanship, public speaking, and interpersonal skills. These courses are popular to this day. He is the author of the bestseller How to Win Friends and Influence People (1936), which is recommended reading for anybody playing the Man/Woman game. Dale Carnegie is an American legend whose practical, down-to-earth ideas on relationships and communication have influenced millions.*

There are no models, as Manson points out, for becoming an attractive and integrated man in the 21st century. Men yearn for a way of life that combines their passion to excel by becoming fully themselves, with their love and desire for women. If that describes you, here is what I suggest: *own your truth.* You are a man who loves women, and who wants them. You simply need to learn to express that, and be that, in a way that works for both you and your partners. In other words, be prepared to do your work. A masculine person must lead in communication. This book will show you how.

This book is one of the very few men's attraction books that work well even at the relationship stage (after the seduction stage), and it is the *only* men's attraction book that even mentions the topic of sacred sexuality, or Tantric sexuality [David Deida, Chris Menné]. Sacred sexuality is something you *will* want to try, but knowing where to begin is difficult. This book will help you with that, and also will guide you through the vast sea of misinformation that surrounds even ordinary human sexuality and the psychology of attraction.

This is the book I wish my father had given me. It would have saved me 10 years in my developmental journey. It would have avoided a great deal of loneliness and hurt that I dealt both myself and my intimate partners during 55 years of living, hurt that was caused by ignorance, and it would have brought me to power much sooner in my life. My ardent hope is that it does this for you.

I will make you a bold promise: if you take on and start practicing these principles in your life whenever the need arises – for instance, when you are having an argument with your partner, or when you are asking a woman out – *you will have results that will greatly surprise you, by becoming a more loving person, one who is naturally more attractive to the opposite sex.*

> ### MARK MANSON (1984 - )
>
> *Manson is a young American author, entrepreneur, personal development and dating coach.*
>
> *His 2011 book Models is a breakthrough in men's attraction literature, and entirely fulfills Manson's stated goal of providing "a model for being an attractive, integrated man in the 21st century." Models is a must-read book for men who wish to understand how their sexuality and the psychology of attraction can fit in to a holistic developmental strategy for themselves.*

And it is even possible that you could make yourself, and at least one woman, *deliriously happy.* I am not young any more, but I am young enough to believe that happiness, or at least being at peace with ourselves and the world as it is, is our human birthright. For many people, deep sexual intimacy is the fastest way to happiness and success. And it could even take you all the way to a spiritual awakening (see Chapter 33).

Many people are strongly motivated to achieve real sexual intimacy. But nobody taught us how to relate powerfully to the opposite sex. Good sexual loving is one of the most profound and most fulfilling of human experiences. Don't give up too soon! It is a lot easier than most people realize.

## Be optimistic: your future is bright

Despite the enormous economic, cultural, political and environmental challenges that the world is facing today, and despite the sexual and emotional misery that many men and women endure, I remain an optimist. You might consider also becoming one.

The reason for my optimism is that I believe that the time has come to *"let us see now what love can do"* [William Penn]. For sure, people have been trying this throughout human history, on and off, but we have never, ever before had the intellectual and material resources, and the freedom, and the network, that we have today. We have reached critical mass, and the phenomena described in this book are going to start to happen, really fast, perhaps even within the next generation.

The fastest way to learn how to love is with our opposite-polarity partners. It is both extraordinarily effective and not that difficult once you get the basic idea, and most men are highly motivated to it. Once you and your woman start to deeply love each other, your love will expand of its own

> **WILLIAM PENN (1644 – 1718)**
>
> *William Penn was an early Quaker (follower of George Fox) and the founder of the state of Pennsylvania, USA. Penn inherited Pennsylvania as a gift that the British King gave to his father. Penn was a visionary for democracy and religious freedom, and created Pennsylvania, and especially the city of Philadelphia, as a utopia, advocating for ideas that were before his time, including equality for women. The results of this experiment are controversial, but it still gives Philadelphia its nickname, "the city of brotherly love".*

accord. Learning how to have real love in your life gives you a critical role in the evolution of human consciousness. Healing relationships between men and women, and re-opening our natural flow of sexual loving, may be the most effective strategy to putting humanity back on the path of love.

***Here is why it is so effective:*** You can stand with your lover in the crucible of creation, the source of life and of all manifestation, you and your lover as a microcosm of the eternal interplay of masculine and feminine. You will be Shiva, dancing with Shakti and creating the world. How this works is a great mystery, a force beyond words and conceptualization, it is the Godhead in each of us. Real love taps into the most powerful force in the Universe. Why not "see what love can do?". indeed.

In other words, playing a sexual polarity game, either externally (the **Man/Woman game**) or internally as described in Chapter 34, could take you closer to the realm of perfect manifestation. This is when the Universe aligns with you without any effort. It is when you barely have to say something, and it happens, often within 24 hours. Many people have experienced this at some time in their lives, whether or not they can explain it.

All of this might strike you as "New Age woo-woo." I am actually an engineer and not usually disposed to such nonsense, but I need to say it. It is possible that it is true. You will need to judge for yourself – after you have been practicing love for a while. Maybe a short while. *"Love is not time-bound"* [Jerry Jud].

## A few disclaimers

First, please translate the terms "man/woman" and "masculine/feminine," into your own particular "gender-speak." We are discussing a relationship style that some people call the **Man/Woman game,** also known as **Sexual Polarity**. It relates to many types of human interactions, and you may find the ideas apply to you regardless of your gender preferences, relationship style, or fetishes. Some more caveats on sexual polarity are offered at the end of Chapter 5.

Second, this book focuses mostly on the masculine side of the Man/Woman game. If you are primarily feminine, you might still find the ideas and practices valuable; but you may also want to look up Alison Armstrong's QUEEN'S CODE, which is a rather precise feminine-polarity counterpart to this book. Alison has, God bless her, built a significant education platform and offers interactive workshops as well.

Third, these ideas are radical, and maybe challenging. Indeed, they are in direct opposition to the dominant relationship model that most Western-educated people have adopted for the last 40 years (see Chapter 20: Feminism and the rise of **Whole and Complete**.)

## An important caveat: the limitations of human developmental systems

Before we begin, let's set realistic expectations: No relationship model, or developmental system whether it deal with sexual polarity or not, will either guarantee success in relationship, or fully model a topic as rich, as deep, as diverse as human relationships.

Learning to love well – with our sexual partners, friends, children, and co-workers – is going to be a lifetime of work. Understanding the fundamentals of good human sexual loving will only account for 10% to 20% of your success, at best. The remaining 80% to 90% you will need to acquire from other teachers and from the school of hard knocks. You will need to be *"wounded in your understanding of love"* [Khalil

**KHALIL GIBRAN (1883 – 1931)**

*Gibran was a Lebanese artist, poet, and writer, best known for his book* **THE PROPHET** *(1923), from which many of his quotes in this book are taken. His writings are heavily influenced by Sufism, a mystical tradition characterized by an emphasis on the ecstatic nature of man's relationship to God. He is the third best-selling poet of all time, behind Shakespeare and Lao-Tsu.*

Gibran]. Eventually, you may need to break all models and structures and just give yourself to love. In the meantime, however, you will likely get hurt, and still you will have a glorious life. There is no way to learn how to love, except by being hurt. It is God's plan, resistance is futile.

Even so, what you can learn in these pages is an *excellent beginning*. And so:

## Let us begin… or at least let us start again

This book is short, and this is by design. I have attempted to write a love manual for men, and so I have taken out the fluff. We men like to get to the point, I hope you will not be disappointed. You can read it all in one sitting, or you can graze by reviewing the topics that currently interest you.

Take a chance with me. Give this book a few hours of your time. Even 15 minutes might give you something priceless.

# 2 The Problem of Sexual Loving, Part 1

*"Depression is the reward we get for being 'good' " – Marshall Rosenberg*

*"Woman is the natural place of refuge for man" – Dieter Duhm*

In its first draft this book was written as a men's seduction manual. I described the lessons of my 40 years of attempting to understand women, and to relate these personal experiences to the latest research on sexual polarity, human loving, and female orgasm. I wanted to help men have more and better relationships with women. That is still my goal, but it has become larger.

I realized very quickly that you cannot discuss meaningfully the problems of man/woman relationships and sexual intimacy without reference to the larger problem of human development and maturation. And this larger problem of human development cannot, in turn, be discussed meaningfully without reference to the problem of **internalized oppression,** which is the root cause of widespread sexual and emotional misery. Our current sexual misery crosses almost all cultures and socio-economic levels, but it is particularly acute in America. Less than half of Americans are sexually satisfied, and we Americans also have far less sex than people in other countries[1].

> ### DIETER DUHM (1942 - )
>
> *Dieter Duhm is a German psychoanalyst, political activist, and author, best known as co-founder of the intentional community and eco-village Tamera, located in Portugal. One of Duhm's fundamental ideas is that we cannot have peace in the world so long as men and women are at war with each other. Duhm was a leftist political activist for many years. He eventually concluded that most alternative and utopian political movements have failed because of relationships between the sexes. Duhm has written 4 books, including his most famous* **THE SACRED MATRIX.**

*"Internalized oppression"* is a psychological concept that describes how we treat ourselves and other people as we have been treated, both by

---

1   THE 12 MOST SEXUALLY SATISFIED COUNTRIES. Alternet.com, Feb. 2014

our parents and by society. Resolving this issue requires deep inner and outer work. I call it **Growing Up.** A man cannot achieve a deep partnership with a woman unless he is a grown-up. The condition of being a grown-up is the essence of this book, so let me describe now the vision that flows naturally from the fulfillment of that condition.

"Growing Up" means to put oneself into mature relationship with the world. It means to make peace with the world and other people as they are, and to find ways to meet one's inner needs within this imperfect world. It means to form a vision for happiness and to find a way to fulfill it. A lot of recent work [Brené Brown[2], Johann Hari[3]] supports the idea that our deepest human need is for connection, to love and be loved. *As such, the fundamental skill involved in growing up is to create loving partnerships with both men and women.* This is a skill that none of us are taught, few understand, and even fewer practice. I myself spent most of my life going about it in entirely the wrong way.

It is very easy to go about this the wrong way, because it requires a radical re-wiring of some natural human instincts and communication patterns. We are just beginning to understand how deep this work actually goes (In addition to this book, I would point interested people to the work of Dieter Duhm, Marshall Rosenberg, and to my blog, manifesting.net). We are not taught to collaborate, or to seek out and encourage the best in other people, and these skills don't come naturally to us.

Above all, what's required to fully grow up is a complex re-channeling of the rage that many of us, and maybe all of us, feel towards the life that has been handed us. There are few practical models for doing this type of inner work, and few people have accomplished this feat. Our political and economic leaders, at home and abroad, have not done so. One need only open the newspaper to see this, since the outcome of this process is compassion for all living beings, especially one's enemies. As such, the real answer to evil in the world is to ask the oppressors: *"What have they done to you, my child?"* [Dieter Duhm]. First and foremost, we must ask that question of ourselves. How and why are we oppressing people around us, cutting off the life force within ourselves,

---

2   DARING GREATLY: HOW THE COURAGE TO BE VULNERABLE TRANSFORMS THE WAY WE LIVE, LOVE, PARENT, AND LEAD. Brené Brown, 2015

3   THE LIKELY CAUSE OF ADDICTION HAS BEEN DISCOVERED, AND IT IS NOT WHAT YOU THINK. Johann Hari in Huffington Post, Jan. 2015

while shaming and blaming and creating misery for everyone? Who among us can categorically declare they are part of the solution rather than the problem? I invite us all to use the Rudi test: *"The true test of your spiritual success is the happiness of the people around you"* [Swami Rudrananda]. And then to redouble our efforts wherever we fail that test. It's not even for others' sake, but for ours.

Finding happiness requires a vision for the future. It hardly ever occurs by some mystical experience overnight (Eckhart Tolle got lucky). The head and the heart must work together, and over time. It also usually requires a developmental community, a peer group who are aligned and supportive. We are just beginning to create these types of communities. They are fundamental to this work.

In terms of the vision itself, this is for each of us to create. I will tell you my vision. Songwriter Peggy Seeger has put it best: *"That all may live as lovers do."* The relationship between human lovers becomes the prototype for all human relationships, and the issue of human loving, sexual and otherwise, becomes part of a public conversation, not relegated to the therapist's office and the bedroom. *Sexuality is a social problem.*

You cannot divorce the problem of human loving from the problem of sexuality. We have tried to do this for thousands of years, and have failed. Most modern attempts at community fail for this very reason. The problem of human loving and human sexuality can, and must, become a group conversation. Jesus was right: **individual happiness cannot be achieved until all are happier.** If the desired outcome is happiness, then truly loving our fellows, *all of them* beginning with our sexual partners and moving on to our enemies, is the only rational action. Until this happens, the best we can hope for is to sigh with relief that we are so much better off than so-and-so, imagine that we can take credit for it, and distract ourselves with the toys and perks of our supposed success. *What kind of happiness is that?*

That is the main problem facing humanity today. All other problems are derivative because until we become conscious of what we really want, until we have plumbed the depths of our anger and outrage at the condition of our lives and of our loved ones – while simultaneously appreciating the potential for healing and joy that lies within our most secret longings and fantasies – until we have done this, we are not free. We can't even act rationally in our own best interests. We fail to understand that *"When we are angry, killing people is too superficial"* [Marshall Rosenberg].

What we really want is to love and be loved, to be seen, to feel safe, to have a genuine opportunity to contribute to others; and until we have aligned our lives around this fundamental goal, there can be little return in terms of true happiness and real human progress. We need to clear up our internalized oppression, the unconscious structures of fear, violence, and shame that we have inherited, structures that cut-off pleasure and love, and hence, tragically, even our capacity for healing. We need

> ### MARSHALL ROSENBERG (1934-2015)
>
> *Rosenberg is the founder of Non-Violent Communication (NVC). His books have sold more than one million copies and have been translated into more than 30 languages. NVC training is now offered in 60 countries and has impacted hundreds of thousands of people. NVC is, on the surface, a communication model for resolving conflicts between people, but it is much more than that. It is an attitude and a set of communication tools designed to evoke, express and fulfill human needs – and particularly needs for closeness, trust, authenticity, and vulnerability.*

to distinguish who we really are from the person that we have been told we should be, that we ourselves believe we should be, and from the knee-jerk ways that we respond to other people – responses that guarantee our needs will not be met. But when that distinction is finally felt, when the oceans of tears have been shed and we have become alive again, when we can respond to others with compassion regardless of how they behave, then we will have little to fear and nothing to be ashamed of. How can we be ashamed for the way we were made? We had nothing to do with it.

We resist the conversation for wholeness, all of us. One of the fundamental reasons, in addition to internalized shame, is that *we resist seeing ourselves through the eyes of others.* We resist feedback (see Chapter 14). Feedback is painful because it challenges our egoism, insecurities, and false self-concept. But beyond that pain lies an unimaginable peace and happiness. I know this. Everybody who has ever had a moment of true intimacy, or who has ever loved, knows this.

This book is my contribution to the conversation. It has been a 30-

year work, in which I have brought together many different strands of research and modern thinking. Some of these ideas have never been published before; Victor Baranco, for example, has not entered the world stage despite his genius. Same for Jerry Jud, and, to a lesser extent, Dieter Duhm. David Deida is popular, and rightly so, but his ideas become even more powerful, and more compelling, within the system that I am presenting.

I hope you find these ideas both intellectually satisfying and practically useful. I hope you will find here a men's relationship and seduction guide that is not merely useful, but transformational.

---

### VICTOR BARANCO (1934 – 2002)

*Victor Baranco was the founder of an intentional community called the Lafayette Morehouse. It is based in Lafayette, California and is still operating. When Baranco died in 2002, leadership of the community passed on to his second wife, Cindy. Baranco is most famous for first demonstrating a woman in orgasm for one hour by way of manual stimulation of the clitoris. Beyond that, he developed a curriculum around group living, communication, sensuality, and man-woman relationships, and created concepts and practices that are as powerful and relevant today as they were 40 years ago.*

---

# 3 The Nature of Personal Power

*"We can choose to be audacious enough to take responsibility for the entire human family. We can choose to make our love for the world be what our lives are really about. Each of us now has the opportunity, the privilege, to make a difference in creating a world that works for all of us. It will require courage, audacity, and heart. It is much more radical than a revolution – it is the beginning of a transformation in the quality of life on our planet. You have the power to 'fire the shot heard around the world.'" – Werner Erhard (quoting Ralph Waldo Emerson)*

The word *"power,"* especially in connection with the word *"love,"* evokes a negative visceral reaction from some people. In response, I ask you to define *"power"* as simply **the power to make a difference in other people's lives, and the power to choose happiness,** even amidst the challenging and distressing aspects of life. Choosing happiness requires **accepting ourselves and other people as they are,** rather than how we want them to be, or how we think they should be.

We will return to this basic idea of accepting ourselves and other people as they are many times. It is the secret of happiness, *and* of success in relationships.

---

### *WERNER ERHARD (1935 - )*

*Werner Erhard is the founder of the transformational program "EST," which became Landmark Worldwide LLC in 1991 after Erhard retired from leadership in order to write and teach on his own.*

*Landmark produces many programs, including the Landmark Forum, one of the most successful transformational programs in the world, with over a million graduates.*

*Concepts from Landmark and from Werner Erhard are woven throughout this book, including the idea of a "distinction," "finding people right," "making a difference," and more.*

---

None of us is granted the ability to choose happiness by default. We must work at it. Very few people were ever taught this. Some of us fall along in the way, and then, tragically, never get up. Others are too frightened to begin. But to follow this path to the end is a glorious journey, the *"Hero's journey"* [Joseph Campbell]. It is rewarding beyond belief. And it is not as difficult as you might imagine. Indeed, life itself is pushing us towards it, whether we want to or not (see Chapter 34). We really have no choice but to play. Our only choice might be to play well, or to play badly.

***The journey to power is the journey to emotional maturity.*** It is also the journey towards deeper forms of relationship, and towards making our love for the world what our lives are about, as in Werner Erhard's quote.

# 4 The War Between the Sexes

*"Men are dumb, and women are mean." – Victor Baranco*

*"Men are afraid that women will laugh at them. Women are afraid that men will kill them." – Margaret Atwood*

In this chapter and the next one, we will start to distinguish the issues that stop men and women from getting along. There are two issues, fundamentally: unhealed hurt, and ignorance. *Unhealed hurt is another name for internalized oppression.*

I am talking mostly to men in this book because men, with their natural leadership qualities, single focus, courage and vision, honesty and depth, loyalty, intelligence and heartfulness, have the capacity to lead us all into love. However, this chapter ends with a direct appeal to women – the first, and last appeal to women I will make. I will then return to speaking to men.

## Men are genetically programmed to support women, take care of them and attempt to make them happy

Men are genetically programmed to support women, take care of them and attempt to make them happy. Now, I am not an anthropologist or evolutionary biologist, so I will pass on the scientific justification for this idea. Just consider this: throughout most of human history, 600,000 years or so, women have carried the power to perpetuate our genes – or not. Is it any wonder that we want to please them?

In the wonderful book **Sex at Dawn,** the authors present some evidence that within the earliest, hunter-gatherer nomadic societies, women retained the power to choose their mates. However...

## The adoption of agriculture changed everything

According to **Sex at Dawn**[4], the adoption of agriculture changed all that, through the need for standing armies and higher levels of social organization. Standing armies became necessary to defend territory and

---

4 **Sex at Dawn: How We Mate, Why We Stray, and What it Means for Modern Relationships.** Christopher Ryan and Cacilda Jetha, 2012.

the stored harvest of food. Prior to this, there was no need to defend territory. If a tribe encountered resistance or hostility, it moved on. Food was plentiful and population scarce, why fight? Higher levels of social organization came about from the need to recruit that army, as well as questions of property ownership, taxes, tithes, etc.

We can easily imagine what happened next.

When societies organized into hierarchies, one of the first things that men did was to restrict, or entirely eliminate, women's power to choose their mates and to grant (or revoke) sexual favors. Why did men do this? Well, first of all because they could, at long last, control women's sexuality; and secondly because they were, well, dumb-ass guys in the area of sexuality, then as now. Women's sexual freedom was inconvenient for men at best, and infuriating at worst – then as now.

The problem of course, is that you cannot legislate intimate relationships, and having sex with an unhappy or angry woman is really not fun. Even the most brutish guy knows this. It's doubly so when she is cooking for you and raising your children. It doesn't matter what kind of social customs, peer pressure, economic dependence, or legislation you enact: women have the power to make men's lives a heaven or a hell, and they always have. Men live for the company of happy, turned-on women who they care for and respond to, and who return the favor tenfold through their happiness, appreciation of us and the *"magnification of love"* [David Deida], which is women's genetically programmed function. This is the **Deep Feminine,** which men live and die for. But when our women are not happy, we men pay. We pay through the **Dark Feminine** and a thousand other ways (see Chapter 23). There is just no winning that game.

> ### DAVID DEIDA (1958 – )
>
> *David Deida is a popular American author, Tantra master and sexual educator. He is the author of more than 10 books translated into 25 languages, including his most famous* **THE WAY OF THE SUPERIOR MAN.**
>
> *Deida has inspired thousands of men and women to greater honesty, authenticity and integrity with their partners, and is a profound influence on me.*
>
> *Read his semi-autobiography* **WILD NIGHTS** *for an entertaining account of the education of a Tantra master, and see the Bibliography for a critical review of his work, and also the chapter on Masculine Purpose.*

Attempting to control women and women's sexuality is a losing game, because women's sexuality is the source of life and, indirectly, of all manifestation. It must be obeyed, not controlled. Even women can't control it. Any attempts to control it will create havoc, which is exactly what has been happening. Trying to control women's sexuality has to be the craziest thought that ever entered into any man's brain.

Consequently, men lost the war between the sexes. Well, obviously, everybody lost. But being dumb-ass guys, not knowing any better and quite preoccupied with survival and reproduction and the creation of civilization, they did nothing until the 20th century, when women finally took back their reproductive rights in much of the world.

However, this did not make the women happy because it is only part of what women want. Women want their men to be happy, successful, self-expressed and powerful, as much as the reverse. The problem is that hardly anybody knows how to relate powerfully to the opposite sex. *Our parents did not teach us, because they did not know.*

Women take responsibility for their own happiness and fulfillment, and the happiness and fulfillment of their men, by enrolling their men into partnership with them. It is a powerful feminine gift to enroll people and find agreement, but few women are ready or able to do this work. Other women are simply not yet willing or able to let go and forgive the last 10,000 years of oppression, invalidation, murder, and rape – which continues to this day.

Now this is not so easy for women, otherwise, they would have already done it, surely. However, the job needs doing. And it's the men who need to take charge here. Women cannot do it alone.

**And yet, for the first and last time in this book, a direct appeal to women:**

Women: *"Lay down your sword"* [Alison Armstrong]. *It's lonely from in here. We miss you... a lot.* We are very sorry for what we did to you in the past, and what some men do to you even now, but how much longer are you going to punish us? How much longer are you going to withhold your love? What is your plan? Do you have a plan? It's not just your happiness that is at stake now, and ours, it is the survival of the species.

And also: only about half of the women of the world (at most) have real sexual freedom, to this day. Despite great improvements in women's freedom in the last century, the gain is only relative.

And so: *Women: what about your sisters who have not yet achieved their sexual freedom – do you care for them?* And if you do, are you willing to *"let us see now what love can do?"* [William Penn]. It took you 150 years to gain sexual freedom in the Western world. Would it not be nice now to free your remaining sisters, but faster and more pleasurably than the first time... and to a far more satisfying result, which is that men would be by your side again, strong and powerful and loving, such as you like them to be?

Enough said. The rest of this book is for men who desire to *"see now what love can do."*

# 5 The Problem of Sexual Loving, Part 2

*"Human beings were made for ecstasy." – Jerry Jud*

**Ignorance** is the second fundamental issue in the way of men and women getting along. We can start to imagine what can be done about it.

## Why are human relationships so difficult?

Ask yourself this: Why are human relationships – and particularly relationships between the sexes – so difficult?

So many men want, more than anything else, the companionship of a loving, creative, sexy woman who respects him, enjoys and appreciates him for who he is, and fills his life with fun, love and adventure... and some men want *only* that.

And so many women want, more than anything else, the feeling of being seen, appreciated, loved and cherished by a man, one whom she feels has his full attention on her when she needs him and is emotionally available... and perhaps a few women would be satisfied with *only* that, while many more would find it an *excellent beginning*.

So given all this: why is there so much anger, loneliness, and misunderstanding between men and women? Why are we still hurting, traumatizing, sometimes even killing each other?

You would think that we have better things to do than oppress and torture each other, after all these years, yes? Why is the war between the sexes still alive and well? Why has women's liberation failed to deliver true happiness and contentment for women?

These issues appear to be particularly real, and pressing, in America. Why? Why did Mother Theresa nominate the United States as the *"loneliest country in the world?"*

Three fundamental reasons:

- First, we share some fundamental misunderstandings on the nature of human loving.

- Second, we are ignorant of the differences between the sexes... and of how easy it can be to succeed with the opposite sex, thereby getting everything we want and more, while spreading love, light and understanding all around us.

- Third, we are lazy in our loving. Yes: *lazy, and stingy.*

So let us begin to clear up some of these misunderstandings.

### The nature of human loving

Psychiatrist Scott Peck wrote a seminal book called **THE ROAD LESS TRAVELLED** (1978). It has inspired millions of people to clarify their values and attempt to live a more loving life. Peck's ideas, along with Jerry Jud's **Skills and Principles of Loving** (see Chapter 8), are part of the primary source material for this book.

Let's begin with Scott Peck's and Jerry Jud's definition of *"real love."*

Forget about love as a feeling. Forget about being in love, or the Hollywood version of the

> **SCOTT PECK (1936 – 2005)**
>
> *Scott Peck was an American psychiatrist and author, best known for his book* **THE ROAD LESS TRAVELLED***, published in 1978. The Road Less Travelled is a profound essay on the nature of human development and maturation, including chapters on love, discipline, suffering, grace, and more. Peck spent his later years developing models of authentic human community and leading workshops designed to create this type of community. These ideas are described in his other major book,* **THE DIFFERENT DRUM.**

love between a man and a woman, also known as romantic love, or infatuation. As pleasurable as it is, pursuing this type of love is rarely a good strategic choice. It also doesn't last long, 18 months at most for many couples... and 24 hours for others. It's also self-serving and a prime candidate for betrayals. It is exclusive rather than general. It is actually not love at all, for the most part. It just feels good for a while. And then it starts feeling awful – at which point you have the choice to transform it into **real love,** or else you move on to another partner and risk spending the rest of your life in pursuit of a sexual or romantic high endlessly repeating the cycle until you die of exhaustion, still unhappy.

*Real love is very simple: it is reaching out to another person in order to serve them, fill a need, or cause them to grow or develop in some way* [Scott Peck and Jerry Jud]. Love in this context is action and intention. It is an *event* that happens between a "lover" – a person who has a momentary surplus of attention or resources – and a "beloved" – a person who has a need for attention, internal clarity, affirmation, or resources. *Real love is an event* – one that leaves at least two people fulfilled and happier for the experience. Studies have shown that just *witnessing* an act of love between other people makes a person happy[5]. Real love is one of the most satisfying and most fulfilling of human experiences. Not to mention, it is free, requiring only your time and attention and your willingness to reach out. And to make the offer more compelling, sexual ecstasy can be a by-product.

> ### JERRY JUD (1920 – )
>
> *Jerry Jud is a Methodist minister who founded the Shalom Mountain Retreat Center in Upstate New York in 1976. He ran the center until his retirement in the early 90's. Shalom Mountain has inspired and transformed thousands of people to become more fully alive through the creation of intentional loving community and the practice of the Skills and Principles of Loving.*

Going into a deeper distinction now, this type of love might also be described as "outer love" or "reaching out." It is only one type of love. *Reaching out is the masculine side of love.* This one-sidedness is at the source of our cultural confusion. *Real love has two parts.*

The other type of real love is *"reaching in," the feminine side of love.* Mature feminine love looks within and finds peace and joy in everything it meets, sees the perfection of all manifestation. It transmutes all experiences and internal events into meaning, especially the hard and difficult emotions, and it does so by accepting them and people as they are. Feminine love is simply self-acceptance and along with it, other-acceptance – radical self-acceptance and forgiveness, including all our own imperfections. It is the unconditional commitment to being happy and to finding purpose and meaning in a world of chaos and cruelty. It is a high and beautiful road to travel.

These ideas are simple, yet infinitely complex in execution. There are

---

5 PRACTICING ACTS OF KINDNESS. Psychology Today, Nov. 2012

also a number of additional, and essential practical distinctions that are covered in Chapter 8.

## Human loving and sexual polarity

The idea of a masculine and feminine side of love, or **Sexual Polarity,** was pioneered by author and Tantra master David Deida. We go into this topic in Chapter 9, but here is a quick summary. This is the 30,000-foot overview.

Imagine for a moment that men and women have a preferred sexual polarity – a way of being in the world and a way of processing their experiences that is going to be different, whether they choose a masculine or a feminine polarity.

And then imagine that most (but not all) men have a preferred masculine polarity, while most (but not all) women have a preferred feminine polarity.

And then consider this idea: most people want to love in the way that matches their polarity – in other words, masculine people prefer outer love (reaching out), and may become skilled at this, while feminine people prefer inner love (reaching in), and may become skilled at this.

And so, what if men and women loving each other well in this way turned out to be a perfectly complementary expression – what if it created a wonderful balance, a naturalness in relationship and a satisfaction and joy that all parties ultimately prefer?

## Please imagine a new world

*Please imagine a world of men in support of women.* It is a type of servant leadership, with men having real attention on women, understanding and supporting the feminine values (fundamentally, *pleasure and love*), and responding to women's needs by using men's natural masculine skills and values of *production and assertion* in the service of women.

And then imagine that the women felt so cared for, seen, and nurtured by this, that they became able to *make an internal decision to be happy no matter what.* And that thanks to this showering of attention and devotion from the men in their lives, and to this internal decision, imagine that they naturally expanded to their fullest capacity and deepest feminine purpose, which is the **magnification of love** [David Deida]. Imagine women becoming so loving, so generous, so appreciative of their partners, so full of life and fun to be around, so beautiful and radiant that they also became *extremely sexual*...

Now, supposing that this dream was to come true: do you think that everyone would be happier? Might there be a lot less fighting between men and women, and more good loving? Would a lot more work get done, and with more pleasure and flow? Would our children be better cared for, our workplaces more appreciative and productive, our politics less adversarial, our communities more vibrant?

This is the key idea of this book. It is not my idea. I have merely integrated a number of different teachers who say similar things, and articulated a program to make it happen. You will see, in the following chapters, how it works. It will all become very clear, I hope. And from there, you will only have to practice.

**It could be the most profound thing you ever do for yourself, and for your partners.**

I dream of an end to the war between the sexes and an end to patriarchy as we know it. What foolishness to dream this!

And yet... I do dream it.

And it is not my dream alone.

Dream with me, and let's see what can happen.

## A note about Sexual Polarity

When we describe someone as being a person of *"masculine polarity,"* or of *"feminine polarity,"* we are talking about a lot more than genitalia, in a multi-layered system that is not binary (true/false). Our **Sexual Polarity** is actually the sum of our individual location on a number of scales. These scales begin with the obvious, our external genitalia, but even at this most basic physical level people do not divide neatly into categories – let alone on the emotional and psychological scales.

In addition to external genitalia, we must also consider the person's sexual orientation, their preference for men or women partners, same-polarity or opposite-polarity partners within that group, dominance/submission, all of these or none, etc. Furthermore, none of the above says anything about a person's gender presentation through clothing, gesture, and mannerisms, which may or may not reflect their internal self-image of themselves as "man" or as "woman," and which may have nothing to do with the flavor of partner they prefer. All of these paths and needs are valid. There is not even any such thing as "normal" in human sexuality, or even a fixed response over time in a single person. The range of sexual needs and expression exceeds even the extraordinary variability of human types and personalities. This is partly why it is so difficult to get it right, and why many of us suffer so much in this area. Assumptions and models all fail at some point.

For these reasons, any concepts relating to a person's dominant sexual polarity must be taken with a large grain of salt. Some even go so far as to reject all human developmental models and even the usefulness of the words "masculine" and "feminine". This is true for them – remember human beings are different and therefore need to be loved differently – but for most of us, this degree of extremism would be "throwing out the baby with the bath water". My advice is to *take what you like and leave the rest* from these ideas, and to apply a good dose of critical intelligence. **Above all, try out these ideas and see if they work for you.** Almost all people respond well to the practices and communication tools I will be presenting – regardless of any conceptual models or words we choose for convenient understanding or intellectual elegance.

# 6 Supporting Women vs. Being a Servant

*"Men without women tend to be flat, predictable and outwardly destructive; women without men tend to be unfocussed, emotionally self-indulgent and inwardly destructive." – David Deida (paraphrased)*

### Men were created for women – but many men resist this idea

This chapter will clarify the meaning of *"supporting and caring for women,"* and also of negative feedback. We cover the topic of women's negative feedback to men in Chapter 14. This chapter begins to look at men's negative feedback to women.

It is difficult for many men to accept and embrace the idea that their natural, genetically programmed function is to support, care for, and respond to women's needs. Perhaps they imagine that to do this means to submit, or lose their power and individuality to women. Perhaps they think of "support and care for" as in "servant" – an endless set of boring tasks, and for no pay, or at best, inconsistent pay.

But the truth is the opposite in every way: ***Supporting and caring for women is actually the fastest way to men's power and to the full discovery and expression of men's individuality.*** The work of supporting women is infinitely varied, delightful, and usually spot-on for the masculine appetites, and the pay is beyond anything that most men can imagine. Caring for women is not just a job, it is men's greatest joy and the fulfillment of their destiny. Men's deepest need is to love, in an active way.

The distinction between *"supporting"* and *"being a servant to"* is simple: ***You are not required to do anything that she asks of you!*** You feed back to her your feelings, and negotiate until it feels right to both of you. You may need to say, *"Let's talk about this, why do you want this, what is the deeper need behind this?"* You may also say *"Alright, but let me think about it."* *"Thinking about it"* means that you will sit on it until you have perfect internal alignment and you have devised a workable plan (or created a **Structure**, see Chapter 34) to make it happen. You may ask her for help here, but if you can't get internal alignment, or figure out a workable plan, you will need to negotiate with her. *Once the two of you are in full alignment, chances are that what she wants – no matter how high the bar – will manifest quickly.*

Reaching full alignment is the goal. Indeed, a man should never do anything for a woman that does not feel right for him, or that doesn't give him satisfaction or a sense of accomplishment in some way. *She is depending on you not to do that. If you did that, you would betray her.* More on this in Chapter 21: Masculine Terms.

### So why do men resist the idea of supporting and taking care of women?

There is one more reason why men resist the idea of supporting women. *Men are brought up to believe that they are better than women.* Men are, with few exceptions, arrogant and full of themselves in relationship to women. We fear, unconsciously perhaps, that if we would agree to *"support"* them, we would be giving up something precious, such as our power to make independent decisions. But what if our real fear is to have to *give up the illusion of our superiority?*

Fundamentally, we think we know better. **Many men believe that we can think better than women, and that women's solutions don't work as well as ours do.**

And this is a tragic error, for two reasons.

First because women's brains, operating as they do in *"diffuse consciousness"* (see Chapter 9), generally have a much more accurate sense of the needs, emotional condition, and capabilities of the people in their environment. By shutting out feminine perspective on the all-important problem of where we men should direct our energy, our time and attention, we are missing out big-time. **We are missing out on the kind of information that can only come from a feminine brain.**

Second because, as has already been stated: achieving deep partnership with women is actually the key to men's power. You are complementing each other's intelligences to obtain a whole that is greater than the sum of the parts. When you become more inter-related and thus more loving, you are, at minimum, doubling your power... and maybe multiplying it by a hundred. You are calling to your aid the most powerful force in the Universe (that would be love). *"Where two or more are united in my name, I am present"* [Jesus].

For sure, you *could* also play the inner game of masculine and feminine exclusively (see Chapter 34), in which case you might not need an external (real-world) woman to partner with. However, because men are genetically programmed to outer love, most men will want a flesh-and-blood woman (or women) to reach their highest potential. *"Cherchez la femme" (Find the woman)* [Alexandre Dumas, père].

Wise men and women know this already, as do all great lovers. This is simply how it is.

### Yet another reason why greater inter-relatedness leads to greater power

It has been proven that human beings who are more inter-related are happier, and also live longer[6]. Happier people are naturally more generous, more receptive, kinder and more collaborative – and hence, usually more effective, or powerful. But there is a further reason, coming from systems theory. A system of greater complexity is more adaptable and hence more resilient. This is particular true of human systems. The path to power in a complex world is through greater inter-relatedness, or collaboration. When we operate more collectively, concerned with other's well-being in addition to our own, loving each other and giving kind and honest feedback, we compensate for each other's blind spots, or developmental gaps. This results in our making better and wiser decisions.

There are even more reasons why collaboration between men and women generates power, reasons that are buried deep in the mystery of creation. We return to this topic in Chapter 35.

---

6   Read anything by Martin Seligman and the Positive Psychology movement, in particular the book **Authentic Happiness**.

## PART 2: FOUNDATIONS

In this part, we lay down the intellectual foundations for the work of loving women: Dieter Duhm and the culture of lying; Jerry Jud and the problem of human loving; and David Deida and Victor Baranco on sexual polarity.

# 7 We Live in a Culture of Lying [Dieter Duhm]

*"It is outrageous when you think about the effort we make to appear different to others than we really are." – Dieter Duhm*

*"The love between man and woman is one of the most beautiful things that one can experience on our Earth. Nobody who is in this state of love can imagine that it will ever be over. Nevertheless, almost all love relations fail. Human society has a collective heartache. For most people, the area in which they could have the most beautiful experiences is an area of deep disappointment, deep suffering, deep anger and often ultimate resignation." – Dieter Duhm*

The discovery of authentic relationship and authentic sexual expression is, for most of us, a personal event of cataclysmic proportions. You will likely feel a fundamental change in your life's purpose and direction. You may drop all your old friends and find new ones, change careers, move, engage new interests and groups, start traveling, experiment with new ways of life, etc. You may go through all kinds of emotional states in the process, from elation to depression and maybe even despair. It is useful, in beginning this journey, to have a realistic assessment of the obstacles you will be facing. **You need to realize that in the journey to becoming an authentically loving, self-expressed and sexual human being, you may not get a lot of support from the culture and from people in your immediate environment.**

You may wonder: why is this so difficult? Why must we humans struggle so much to find happiness and love? And why do we continue to do such terrible things to each other, using both bullets and words to devastating effect? The answer is complex, and is partly buried in the mystery of creation. The battle between good and evil, between love and fear, seems to be part of the fabric of the universe, an aspect of God's plan for human re-emergence, what some call the "atonement" [Course in Miracles].

But beyond the existential fact of the universality of suffering, *there is also the fact that Western culture and religious institutions have been waging a war for thousands of years against sexuality, against women, against human diversity, and against the full expression and fulfillment of some of our deepest human needs.* Dieter Duhm calls this "the rape of love" -- meaning that the world's institutions have systematically and brutally attempted to destroy some of the deepest and most important aspects of our humanity, beginning with sexuality. They have justified this destruction in the name of morality – a false morality. *A morality that does not support love is, by definition, a false morality.* We all carry the imprint of this war, and it throws numerous obstacles in the way of our search for a happier and more loving way of life.

*The outcome of Western culture's war against sexuality is internalized oppression.* This chapter discusses its origins and our usual response.

## Our culture does not encourage us to express and then go after our deepest needs

Our culture does not encourage to go after our deepest wants and needs. In fact, it barely recognizes them at all. Instead, it tells us what to want – and most of the time, we believe these stories. We try really hard to find happiness and fulfillment by living the life we are told we should live and by procuring the things that we are told we should want. And since this rarely works, many of us are reduced to the "life of quiet desperation" [Henry David Thoreau].

***The most direct result of this cultural programming, is that we lie constantly, to ourselves and others, about what it is that we really want and need*** – or, at best, we fail to speak our entire truth. And the closer the unexpressed want or need gets to the heart of our humanity, the more we lie. *Nothing gets closer to the heart than matters of: love, sexuality, attention, affection, and belonging. So these are the things that we lie about the most.*

## How we internalize cultural oppression

When we receive messages from society and from people in our environment that do not fit our true nature, we do two terrible things. The first terrible thing we do to ourselves, and the second we do to other people. All of us – men, women and children – are both victims and perpetrators of internalized oppression.

***The first thing we do in response to cultural oppression is to imagine***

*that we are the problem.* In other words, we take on the false value or false belief, and attempt to mold ourselves to the ideal which the false belief describes. Remember that the reason false morality is so effective is that it carries a seductive ideal. Maybe we pursue the "American dream" of career and family, but then find ourselves deeply unhappy. We wonder what type of flaw this reveals in us, given that all our peers have accepted this same belief, apparently, and more than likely are coaching us to try harder.

*The second thing we do in response to our cultural oppression is even more cruel: we do to others as we have been done to.* Our parents beat us or shamed us, so we beat or shame our children. We learn that gaining wealth and power is the only way we will get love and attention, and so we kill ourselves in the pursuit of wealth – while treating with contempt people who are poor or struggling. We have learned that "boys don't cry", so when our male friend cries, we turn away in embarrassment. And so on.

*And to make the situation even more tragic, we don't even know that we are doing these terrible things.* We have no awareness of the psychological damage being done to us and by us. We are like fish who do not know they are swimming in water – a toxic water. We know, perhaps, that something is wrong through a vague sense of unease, or maybe even hopelessness and despair; but we do not fully understand the causes. We imagine it is our personal problem. And this prevents us from reaching out honestly to others, which would be the most rapid solution. If we knew, in our hearts, that everyone has the same fundamental problems that we do, we would be much less inhibited in reaching out.

## We are living inside a vast cultural conspiracy of shame and denial around the power and importance of sexual needs

Sexuality is the most critical area of our internalized oppression, because it is one of the deepest human needs. As Dieter Duhm says, the love between man and woman is one of the most beautiful things that one can experience. And yet we are almost all deeply wounded and hurting in this area. To the point that many of us have given up.

*The issue of love is a global issue.* In your search for authentic love and sexual expression, you must not forget that you are taking on Western culture, full-on.  The journey is not for the faint of heart.  *However, it might be the most worthwhile journey.*

We continue now, with important distinctions on human loving and sexual polarity.

# 8 Skills and Principles of Loving [Jerry Jud]

*"More than anything else, we want to love and be loved" – Jerry Jud*

You are going to learn many powerful techniques for relating to people with feminine sexual polarity in this book. But unless you approach these techniques with a good attitude, it is quite probable that you will make a bigger mess than when you began. The **Skills and Principles of Loving** are at the core, and it is important to understand them if you are going to succeed. You can practice these skills and principles with a person of any polarity and will likely have great results; but if you practice sexual polarity without understanding the skills and principles you will likely get into trouble.

Before we begin, a caveat: this book is written from a masculine perspective, and some people may find these ideas radical, challenging, and maybe unsettling. Others may find these concepts meaningless or even offensive. Please, keep an open mind, take what you like and leave the rest.

## How the Skills and Principles came about

The **Skills and Principles of Loving** were derived by another beloved teacher of mine, Jerry Jud.

A brief history of Jerry Jud: he was minister to a large Methodist congregation when he noticed that most of the people barely knew each other and were not intimate with each other. He researched this problem and eventually concluded that people cannot be intimate in a structure that denies or represses sexuality. Why? Simple: *because when people become intimate they sometimes develop sexual feelings for each other!* To achieve intimacy with someone, you need a way to channel your sexual energy. If you are repressing or denying your sexuality, it is going to be difficult or impossible to achieve true intimacy.

Jerry Jud discovered that human sexuality is linked to intimacy of any kind, including non-sexual intimacy and the deeper forms of human collaboration. If this is true, it suggests that sexuality is a fundamental driver of all that is fine and wonderful in humans. Throughout the majority of human history, sexuality has often been regarded as some necessary evil at best, and shameful or animalistic at worst. ***How far from the truth, and how tragic.***

Jerry Jud ultimately left his church and founded the Shalom Mountain Retreat Center in New York State in which these skills and principles are practiced by way of residential retreats. Shalom means "peace" in Hebrew, but the center is not otherwise connected to Judaism. Shalom retreats are extraordinarily powerful and quite affordable; if you have the opportunity to attend one, grab it.

Here are the **Skills and Principles of Loving** as taught by Jerry Jud:

### Principles of Loving

- More than anything else, we want to love and be loved.

- Love is a gift.

- Love is not time bound.

- Love is good will in action.

- Love is a response to a need.

### Skills of Loving

- **Seeing**: I do not look over or through you, I see you in your uniqueness.

- **Hearing**: I listen to what you are saying.

- **Honoring of Feelings and Ideas**: I recognize your right to think and feel as you do.

- **Having Good Will**: I will you good and not evil. I care about you.

- **Responding to Need**: If you let me know what your needs are, within the limits of my value system, I will not run away. I will be there for you.

These principles embody four important distinctions.

## Applying the Skills and Principles of Loving: first distinction

**Love is not entirely (or even mainly) a feeling** – it is not something that happens to us. It is an *activity* that involves both outer work (primarily attention and appreciation) and inner work (accepting people as they are and **finding them right** as they are). To love well, according to Jerry Jud, is a lot of work. Nobody is born knowing how to do it. Loving must be learned. We learn how to love by practicing the skills, getting feedback from the people we try to love, and by experiencing people loving *us* – that is, watching them

> **"FINDING PEOPLE RIGHT"**
>
> *This is the ability to find something to agree with and appreciate with anyone you are interacting with. It is based on the idea that we are products of our genes and of our environment, and it is therefore highly probable that if you were in their shoes you would behave exactly the same as they do. "Finding people right" is Jerry Jud's third skills of loving, also expressed as "recognize their right to think and feel as they do."*

demonstrate love. It's extremely helpful to understand this first basic distinction because it clarifies many misconceptions and false ideas, particularly those surrounding the traditional view of romantic love. Romantic love exists happily within Jud's model, however romantic love is only a small part of the benefit. There is so much more.

The idea that *love is action and intention,* and not primarily a feeling, is very important. It is the keystone of Scott Peck's view as well, in **THE ROAD LESS TRAVELED.** It means that we don't "fall in love" with someone simply because they happen to cross our paths and we like some quality that they have, such as their intelligence, beauty or sense of humor. We don't *fall* in love, we *choose* to love someone.

*But why and when do we "choose to love someone"? Typically, when we believe (or intuit) that we can make a difference to them, or contribute something to their lives.*

### Second distinction of the Skills and Principles

**Love is a response to need.** This genius distinction also was best articulated by Jerry Jud: Our loving response is called out or evoked by the other's need. With no need, there can be no love. Now, without the "choice to love" there also can be no love. But it all starts with a need that we perceive in another person, and which we **choose** to respond to.

***Love happens when we choose to respond to another person's need.***
Their need is what attracts us to them – not their strong and beautiful qualities. What causes us to want to love someone is the possibility that we could be accepted by them and make a difference to them, or could contribute something to their life. This is not always a conscious choice.

Is it possible that human beings are simply going about their lives seeking, actively or passively, consciously or not, an opportunity to love someone and make a difference to them? Could it really be true that "more than anything else, we want to love and be loved"? This is exactly the same idea expressed by Marshall Rosenberg's **NON-VIOLENT COMMUNICATION**: The ultimate human desire is simply to *"contribute to life."* We are here to contribute to other people and to life and when we do, the reward is happiness. It's really that simple.

In Sexual Polarity terms, we might say this: In masculine language, *"making a difference"* to a woman might be called *"winning with her."* *"Winning with her"* is related to giving her what she deeply wants, which is the same as loving her well. This is sometimes called *"knowing how to handle her"* – which can be translated as responding to her objections in a way that is satisfactory to her, or makes her happy, which is also the same as loving her. Hence, men will be attracted to women whom they think they can win with.

> ### MARSHALL ROSENBERG AND NON-VIOLENT COMMUNICATION (NVC)
> *NVC is a communication process developed by Marshall Rosenberg beginning in the 1960s. It focuses on three aspects of communication: self-empathy, empathy, and honest self-expression. The core practice of NVC is to discern other people's needs (listen for the hidden needs that underlie all human communications, even communications that are expressed as demands or judgments) and then express or mirror these needs back to other people with empathy. To do this is one of the greatest acts of love. More information about NVC in Chapter 36.*

In feminine language, making a difference for a man is called *"loving him."* Women will be attracted to men whom they think they can accept, approve of, and love – despite any flaws. And since both sexes enjoy a challenge (up to a point and in some perverse way), the greater the challenge and opportunity to make a difference to a woman by winning with her, or the greater the challenge and opportunity to make a difference to a man by loving and approving of him, the greater will be the attraction. Warning: don't take this literally – women who are playing *"hard to get"* and men playing *"hard to love."* If your goal is love, this won't work. **The essence of the game is authenticity.**

## Returning to needs:

Suppressing and denying needs is deeply ingrained in Western culture. Many people are ashamed of having needs, particularly the kind of needs that we cannot meet for ourselves – and that is the majority of deep human needs. This suppression and denial of needs in our culture, and especially in America, may be the reason that Mother Theresa called the United States the *"loneliest country in the world."* Jerry Jud suggests a different way of looking at the problem of human needs. Human needs are, quite simply, the thing that evokes love. Love is an energetic exchange between two people in which both lover and beloved are fulfilled. But without the need, whether it be expressed directly by the receiver, or simply intuited by the giver, love will not happen. *Ergo: needs are good! They are the fundamental driver of the most fulfilling and satisfying thing that you will ever do: loving another human being, or being loved yourself.*

Fully taking on this idea of the critical role of needs as the fundamental driver of human loving might forever change your relationship to your own needs, possibly causing you to become kinder to yourself. Many people have needs they don't understand and might prefer to forget about – even as we guilt and shame ourselves for having them in the first place. Unfortunately the needs persist, and generally get more insistent the more we deny them and wish they would go away.

*Sexual intimacy is one of our greatest needs and the one most frequently repressed and invalidated.* Doubly so as many of us, men and women, often simply repeat the same self-destructive patterns in pursuit of our sexual and relational needs. We do this because nobody ever taught us a different way. And so we follow cultural norms for sexual loving that are broken and lead to poor results. Remember, nobody is born knowing how to love. And we are particularly not born knowing how to love people of the opposite sex. Our parents, for the most part, did not know this either, so give them a break too.

Note that we don't actually have to *"like"* someone in order to *"love"* them. We simply have to *"act lovingly"* towards them. *"You get more points by loving the hard ones"* [Victor Baranco]. When you add the idea that *"love is not time-bound"* – meaning that what might take you little time and effort could have a huge impact on somebody else – then it makes a lot of sense to go about the day with some intention of being more loving. Besides being satisfying in and of itself, being more loving could win you many friends and allies, and might also get you more good sexual loving than you ever dreamed possible.

### Third distinction of the Skills and Principles

**How do we "act lovingly" towards other people?** In principle, it's very simple: We begin by *"acknowledging their right to think and feel as they do,"* also known as *"finding them right."* **We acknowledge their perfection.** We accept that if we were born into their shoes and had their experiences, we would probably behave exactly the same. They are a perfect expression of their genes and of the environment that has nurtured them – including the quality of love that they have been exposed to. So, we don't argue with them that they should think or feel this way or that. We don't tell them that they are wrong to be how they are, or that they are making a mistake. **We assume that they have a good reason for being the way they are, and we try and understand and accept that.**

And from this essential first step, we can extend ourselves to them in an attempt to meet their need. We may listen to them, give them attention, give them feedback and advice if they want it, share our resources with them (food, shelter, money, whatever) – it will all depend on their need. We offer them our acceptance, approval, and encouragement to find their own way, to firm up their value system and become the best they can be inside of that.

The most basic human need, however, is simply attention. *The fundamental act of loving is giving good attention.* And not just any type of attention, but the type of attention people want: **loving attention.**

### Fourth distinction of the Skills and Principles

**I will not run away.** But, you may ask – if we are to go through our lives giving other people all of our attention and all of our resources, how could this work? We would feel constantly drained and not get anything else done.

And this is where Jerry Jud's fourth distinction comes in: *"If you express your needs to me then, within the limits of my value system, I will not run away. I will stay for you (love you)."*

**"Within my value system" is key.** Giving you everything I have until I am left with nothing is outside my value system. Giving you something you want, but which betrays myself, is outside my value system. Giving you something you need but that I don't want to give you or that makes me unhappy or resentful to give you, is outside my value system. We must use great discernment in loving people. Not just in having good attention on them, so that we can accurately predict what they need and then give it to them, but also in terms of taking care of ourselves, so that our own deep well is full most of the time.

## So here are the big problems with human loving

**First problem:** if we accept that the fundamental currency of love is *attention,* then how can we increase our attention without depleting ourselves, or getting nothing else done?

The answer is that we can increase the **quality** of our attention, so that we give the same amount of attention, as it were, in a shorter time (remember, *"love is not time-bound").* So, for example, we try and avoid having repetitive conversations that don't go anywhere, and angry interactions that leave everyone upset. We strive to construct *quality* conversations with people – conversations that make a difference, that transform lives. *"The true test of your spiritual success is the happiness of the people around you"* [Swami Rudrananda].

**Second problem:** becoming a *"good lover"* is quite difficult.

To become a good lover we must grasp the perfection of everyone around us and we must accept them as they are. *"There is a good reason they are the way they are." "Honor their right to think and feel as they do."*

And then, we must attempt to respond to other people accurately in terms of what they really need for their own healing and transformation, which will be different for everyone.

And finally, we must balance all of this with our own needs and self-care.

Becoming a good lover requires a lifetime of learning and of work. It never ends.

## But there is some good news about human loving

- The first good news: The act of loving people can be extraordinarily fulfilling. It is fulfilling in and by itself, of course. But also, when we truly and deeply love other people, by making an effort to extend ourselves to them and care for them, **they very often love us back.**

- The second good news: The styles (or patterns) of loving that most people need are quite predictable. Almost all humans, for example, want quality attention. If you learn to give quality attention, which includes giving people appreciation and acknowledgement, most of your relationships are going to be home runs. It's that simple.

- The third good news: The styles of loving that people want and need tend to be gender-based. Loving a person with masculine polarity can be quite different from loving a person with feminine polarity.

- The fourth good news: You do not have to be an expert to begin. In fact, nobody is an expert. We need only *"love as best we understand love."* We need only have *"faith as small as a mustard seed"* that we are capable of loving people and thereby healing ourselves... and thus the world.

We also need to accept feedback, learn from our mistakes and be humble. When we love people poorly, they will either tell us directly, give us some non-verbal cue, or distance themselves. We need to learn how to see social cues and how to respond to them.

But – we all need to begin this journey, for the sake of the world (the people around us), and just as importantly, for ourselves. And sooner is better than later.

We can play a game described by the poet Khalil Gibran in THE PROPHET:

> *"When love beckons follow him, though his ways are hard and steep...*

*"And when he speaks to you believe in him, though his voice may shatter your dreams as the north wind lays waste the garden…*

*"And think not you can direct the course of love. If it finds you worthy, it will direct your course. Love has no other desire but to fulfill itself….*

*"But if you love and must needs have desires, let these be your desires:*

*"To know the pain of too much tenderness. To be wounded by your own understanding of love. To wake at dawn with a winged heart and give thanks for another day of loving."*

The key here: ***"To be wounded by your own understanding of love."*** Despite our best intentions, we will often fail to love people well. We will carry ideas and assumptions about them that are false. We will be triggered, we may lash out, be selfish and unconscious, project our own stuff on people, and behave in any number of unloving ways.

But it's ok – *if we learn and grow* from our experiences. It is how humans are designed and what is meant to happen. There is, quite simply, no other way.

## In conclusion

For many people, ***sexual intimacy is the fastest and most direct path for learning how to love.*** Why? Well, two reasons:

- The first reason is that sexual intimacy encompasses a significant section of the human experience.

- And the second reason is equally simple: ***we are motivated.*** "Genetically driven" or "compelled" would be more accurate for most of us. When it is not met, sexual intimacy becomes a compelling need for many people. And this is a good thing! Because without it, many of us would not be motivated enough to take on the long, difficult, laborious and sometimes painful task of learning how to love.

Guess what – God has a plan! And it's not a bad one.

# 9 Sexual Polarity [David Deida, Victor Baranco]

*"Women doubt their attractiveness; men doubt their production" –*
*Victor Baranco*

*"The desire to surrender oneself is intrinsic to the sexuality of women*
*and, like everything that is feminine, exists in a smaller extent in men*
*as well" – Dieter Duhm*

## Sexual Polarity According to David Deida

David Deida is another prime inspiration for this book. Deida
popularized the concept of **Sexual Polarity** and has explored the topic
deeply in his books.

Deida suggests that most men will have a primary *"masculine essence"*
and most women will have primary *"feminine essence."* These terms are
defined below. He also suggests, however, that *our sexual polarity is a*
*preference, or choice in the moment.* It can change throughout the day,
and depending on who we are with and what roles we want to play. This
idea is what makes Deida's theory so useful: men and women both can
play from either the masculine or feminine pole. **We are not slaves to**
**our physical gender.**

But despite the fluidity of our sexual polarity choice in the moment, most
of us prefer, and tend to stay, in a single sexual polarity. Men, in particular,
tend to embody a masculine polarity most of the time – meaning they are
generally happier and more productive if they function from a masculine
polarity. If this is true for you, then fully occupying your preferred polarity,
and then finding an opposite-polarity partner to play with in love, in work
and in sex, may be the most direct path to a fully alive, connected, creative,
and satisfying life.

## Why play in the field of Sexual Polarity?

The benefits that you will get by playing in the field of sexual polarity
will likely be in direct proportion to the value (or importance) that you
give to deep emotional connection with people and to sexual expression.
The more you value deep connection, trust, and authenticity, and the

more important is your sexuality to you, the more these ideas will benefit you.

Playing in this field is not just limited to sex, or even to sexual and romantic relationships. It's possible to let principles of sexual polarity, along with the higher-order **Skills and Principles of Loving**, inform your relationships with everyone in your life, man or woman. It's possible that doing this well will lead you to a degree of success in all of your relationships and your career that you would never have dreamed of, to making a big difference in a lot of people's lives, and perhaps even to living a life deeply connected to spirit.

And since one's sexual polarity is a preference and not necessarily an absolute, then *these concepts may apply equally well to gay, lesbian, gender-queer, and transsexual couples* – just substitute your particular gender-speak. They can apply to friendships and work relationships as well.

## Masculine and Feminine processing styles [David Deida]

Now let's briefly consider the nature of your preference between masculine and feminine ways of being.

Many teachers agree that masculine people – which includes most men most of the time, and everyone some of the time – masculine people *prefer a processing style called "single-pointed consciousness."* They are able to focus intensely on a single problem or goal, go deeply into that topic, find out everything there is to know about it, and then design and execute a strategy for success. Single-focus, also known as problem-solving, is the delight of masculine people, and one of their gifts. Deida says **the masculine goal is freedom** – that is freedom from some constraint or from some pain, the resolution of which is the hoped-for outcome. It might also be the freedom of complete awakening or enlightenment. Masculine people, at their best and worst, also have an ability to ignore anything not immediately related to their current single-focus. Including, notably, their partner's needs and emotional states. This is a big problem for women, which we will return to later.

***Feminine consciousness is more inclusive, or less differentiated.***
Feminine people – meaning, people who are relating to the world from a feminine style in the moment – are less concerned with differentiating, judging, or ordering their experiences toward maximizing a pre-

determined outcome. They just take it all in and respond. *"Responding"* to a person or an event is very similar to *"loving"* it. At their best, feminine people love things and people in their environment – meaning they respond to them by valuing them and then possibly transforming them into something even more wonderful, through their love. Feminine people act as **love projectors**. They consume an experience and they magnify or project it into their environment, putting everyone around them into joy and delight. ***The feminine goal is love.***

*To summarize: masculine people try to make life more wonderful by solving problems and/or removing constraints; feminine people try to make life more wonderful by receiving, enjoying, and valuing an experience, thereby multiplying its value and carrying everyone around them into their joy.*

### How to use sexual polarity to your advantage [Victor Baranco]

Once you understand that masculine and feminine people have radically different ways of processing and valuing their experiences, you can begin to leverage these differences to your advantage. You may discover how beautifully complementary these two modes of being are, and the happiness and power that you can gain by understanding these differences and then responding to the needs of your opposite-polarity partner – needs that are going to be quite different from yours. It's not that difficult, and it is a high form of love: responding to a person from where they really are, and not from where you would like them to be or as a mirror of yourself. This is one of the great withholds of human relationships and the secret of many, if not all, happy couples.

If you are a masculine person, you may discover how much better and more satisfying your life can become by allowing your attention – your awesome problem-solving skills and extraordinary differentiation capabilities, also known as **masculine discernment** – to be directed by a wise feminine person's appetite for pleasure and for love. You may achieve a lot more in your life and solve many more and bigger problems – one of the keys to your happiness – and potentially reach a degree of power and success unmatched by people who happen otherwise to be smarter or better connected than you.

If you are a feminine person, you may discover how easily a masculine person's attention can be directed toward your goals. You may discover, indeed, that deep down a masculine person seeks only to care for you and make you happy – and that by allowing him to do this, by trusting him with a kind of authorship for your happiness and assuming he is always doing his best for you, you are helping both of you. This is a complex exchange, and it's not always easy to play it right. But if you assume this exchange as the underlying dynamic of your relationship, and live into it informed by your extraordinary feminine capacity and craving for love, you are both likely to win.

*Here is the value proposition, in its simplest expression:* If you are a masculine person, focusing quality attention on a feminine person is likely to make you happier and more productive. And if you are a feminine person, learning to properly direct a masculine person's focus of attention onto yourself and your goals will not only make you happier, it will also help him too. And what's more, *everyone typically gets better, and/or more frequent, sex.*

Acting and communicating with your opposite-polarity partner in a way that works for them, and meets their deep needs, is the main idea of this book. It is a practice sometimes referred to as **Sacred Sexuality** or **Sacred Intimacy.**

On a practical psychological level this practice works by pooling our very different intelligences towards a common goal – her love and happiness, and his freedom and success. These feminine and masculine goals – love/happiness alongside freedom/success – support and complement each other perfectly. To a large degree they are the same goal, but from different perspectives. We are harnessing the deep power of human sexuality towards greater collaboration, through understanding and valuing gender differences. Understanding gender differences is an aspect of emotional intelligence.

In Chapter 35, we cover more reasons why the practice of sexual polarity can be so extraordinarily effective.

### What is the Man/Woman game – and why play at it?

The **Man/Woman game** is an application of the theory of sexual polarity to a relationship with an opposite-polarity person.

Now, to be sure there are many ways to play in relationship besides what we are discussing here. **Man/Woman** might not be the best game for you, it is probably not even the ultimate game that a man and a woman can play together. Even so, it is a very fine game – and is a particularly good *starting place* for a relationship. Understanding these ideas and practicing them in your relationships could radically transform your life, and make at least two people very happy.

It's true that you could do none of this and still have a great life. However, if you are like most men for whom the love of women is the most profound and compelling experience – and for most women this is even more true – then you would be very foolish not to at least give it a try. **Indeed: If you are a man who likes women, or a woman who likes men, you will ignore these ideas at your peril.**

The next section of this book will offer practical approaches to the problem of relating to an opposite-polarity person, especially a feminine person. We will show you how and why hitching your star to a person or to people with opposite polarity who are right for you is likely to make everyone more powerful and is likely to give you a better life.

# PART 3: BASIC MAN/WOMAN

We build on the theoretical foundations of the previous section, introducing many practical distinctions on what it actually takes to create happy and fulfilling relationships between men and women.  I write from a masculine perspective, but these ideas can be applied profitably by either gender.

If you hope to derive any benefit from this book, approach it as a research project and resolve to practice these ideas. Do your homework, *simply reading will not be enough.* You will need to pick up the phone and call a woman, or else interact with one or more women in a public place. Call her for the sole purpose of appreciating her for how she shows up for you, or what she has done for you. If you can't think of any women to appreciate, call your mother.

# 10 Seduction 101: Women Call, Men Respond [Victor Baranco]

*"We think it is Ok to seduce and 'manipulate' a person for his or her pleasure and welfare." – Steve & Vera Bodansky*

Much of the practical information and distinctions covered in this chapter are derived from Steve and Vera Bodansky's brilliant book, To Bed Or Not To Bed, and in the follow-up book Extended Massive Orgasm. The information presented here is known by all men and women who are successful at the seduction game, and yet, oddly, it has not entered the cultural mainstream. To play the man/woman game successfully, we usually must begin by unlearning everything that we have been taught.

## Women fish; it's the men who are "caught"

The greatest cultural misconception we have relating to the man/woman game is that men are the hunters. In actuality, the opposite is true: women are the hunters – or, more precisely, the fisher-women, who dangle their bait in order to "catch" the men. Men take the bait, or not; but even those who do take the bait must demonstrate their worth or be thrown back into the sea.

The reasons that the seduction game has evolved in this way are many, but fundamentally relate to the fact that, biologically, women have more at stake than men in relationship. As such, women are more selective in the partners they choose. Women create tests for aspiring suitors, hoping that the men will pass these tests and receive the prize of love and sex, which is what everybody wants. Men pass these tests and demonstrate their worth by responding accurately to women's desire, or appetite. To be successful in relationship, men must learn what women want and then give it to them. Women initiate the attraction (or seduction) cycle and they decide on the outcome. Men often make the mistake of pursuing women who are not putting out attraction signals or expressing any real appetite, also known as "heat"; but even when men do respond in some way to feminine desire, they often respond inaccurately and fail the test.

## Women hide their true desires

The game of men providing for women and satisfying their desires is made quite challenging by an additional circumstance: that women hid their true desires, hoping that men will read them and intuitively give them what they want. There are many reasons this is so, but let me cite two. First, women asking directly for what they want would preclude the men showing enough attention and discernment to give the women what they want without being asked, which is what the game is about, a least in the initial stages. Remember, women create selection filters for the men they want to be with, for reasons both biological and cultural. The second reason is that since women are second-class citizens in almost all cultures (not "part of the club") they will not ask directly for what they want for fear of being rejected or shamed. An oppressed group in any culture must, in order to survive, know more about the oppressors than the reverse. In essence, women have been trained for millennia to be men's servants, and the effects of this conditioning still survive. Women are discouraged to go directly after what they want, an especially in matters of sexuality. This is the reason that women have, i general, more real attention and discernment on men than the reverse. Men are, as a rule, clueless in relationship to women until they have been 'caught' and educated by a willing woman in how to please her, and on how to please women in general.

## What women really want; resistance to pleasure; and the push pull game of seduction

Women want many things, different for each woman, of course, and always changing. However, the things that women want generally fit int three broad categories: attention and appreciation; material things; and sex and romance.

The problem of giving women what they want is made even more difficult by two more circumstances. First is the fact that human being and women in particular, are not always clear on what they actually deeply want. And second, all human beings have fear and resistance around the fulfillment of their deepest desires. This is the problem of "havingness", also known as resistance to pleasure.

## "Havingness" for pleasure

Humans tend to live in mood swings of fulfillment and frustration, joy and pain. At any given moment, we can only go as high as we are able to receive, or let go and surrender into pleasure. "Havingness" can be thought of as the upper limit to the pleasure that we can receive in any given moment – regardless of the quality of love and attention being directed towards us.  It can be a permanent limit (i.e. a limit self-imposed by our conditioning), or it can be a temporary limit.  Sometimes, we are just "full".  We have had enough, even enough pleasure. We need to take a time-out and digest an experience before we can fully receive and enjoy the next experience.  It is very important to be tuned-in to people's "havingness" for pleasure when we are relating to them and attempting to respond to their needs.

All human beings want to love and be loved.  The most direct way to provide this experience to people, as discussed in Chapter 9, is to give them attention and appreciation.  This is the most basic and most important human need. In Chapter 12, we go deeply into the ways that you can give women attention. The problem is that people have varying degrees of "havingness" for attention and appreciation. If you give more than they are ready or able to receive, they may resist and even get angry at you and push you away.  Being sensitive to this resistance is fundamental in human relationships, and particularly in the man/ woman game. When you are "too eager to please" and are providing women attention and appreciation that they may not want or are not ready to receive in the moment, you are not loving them well.  You are relating to them out of your needs rather than theirs. You are not truly seeing them for who they are, or honoring their emotional condition. This is a big turn-off in relationship, and will not help your goal of seducing them into pleasure.

## Push people in the direction in which they are already going

It is wise in all relationships, and even more so in the seduction game, to "push people in the direction that they are already going" [Victor Baranco].  This means that if they are already responding to you, then continue what you are doing and maybe even give them more. But if they are not responding, or else they are giving you non-verbal cues that they are not intersted in you, or else have received enough  attention, your best strategy is to honor that and pull back.  You can even push them away: maybe end the conversation, or agree with them by telling them that it's been a fun conversation but that you now have work to do.. This might look like a game, or a manipulation, but it is actually responding accurately to what they want, which is of course an aspect of loving them. It can also be seen as a way to give them an opportunity to come after you, on their own schedule, which might be empowering for them.

The game of seduction is fundamentally a game of push-pull. Of course you want to discern what they really want and give it to them – but maybe not all at once! Give them an opportunity to enjoy your attention and the fact that you may be attracted to them. If you appear too eager to please, however, or "want them too much", they may think that something is wrong with you and become less attracted.

Notwithstanding the above, we live in a culture in which people are so starved for attention and appreciation, that most men most of the time are better to err in the direction of providing too much attention than not enough. Still, use your discernment.

In the next chapter, I will discuss another related and very common problem in relation to women: men's failure in self-investment.

# 11 Self-Investment and the Paradox of Female Sexual Attraction [Mark Manson]

*"Until you learn to trust your own actions and learn to pursue women with your own unique style and personality, you learned absolutely nothing."*

*– Mark Manson*

## Mark Manson's <u>Models</u>

Mark Manson's 2011 book MODELS is a breakthrough in men's attraction and seduction literature. It is a comprehensive dating and relationship guide based on the fundamental idea that for men to attract and then successfully relate to women they need first to *invest in themselves,* and from there to become more discerning, authentic, and vulnerable men. Such men have a higher quality of attention to offer women because they have less attention on themselves. By investing in ourselves, we naturally move into a space of simply wanting to add value and contribute to women. This is both more effective and more fun than traditional seduction techniques, which are often based on salesmanship, that is, giving an *impression* of added value.

Manson's stated goal is to provide a model for being "an attractive, integrated man in the 21st century." He succeeds brilliantly at this goal, with the added bonus that his ideas work for seduction as well.

Men yearn for a way of life that combines their passion to excel by becoming fully themselves, with their love and desire for women. This is, no doubt, why Manson is so popular. MODELS is a must-read book for men who wish to understand how their sexuality and the psychology of attraction can fit in to a holistic developmental strategy for themselves.

Manson provides an acute analysis of modern-day relationships and particularly the dating game, gives innumerable and priceless examples, and gives many attitudes and practices for men to achieve satisfying partnerships with women. In particular, MODELS provides deep insights and advice on the idea of **self-investment**, an idea that is critical to success in relationship, for both men and women.

As Lovers Do extends Manson in the areas of conscious relationship, the theory of sexual polarity, emotional communication, and sacred sexuality. So let's review Manson's fundamental ideas as a starting place to the higher skills of loving.

## Foundations of female sexual attraction

The most puzzling topic of all is the nature of women's sexual attraction. Men have been trying to understand this for millennia, but it is only recently starting to get clear through the theory of sexual polarity and evolutionary biology.

A man's initial attraction to women is *visual*. It is based on a woman's appearance, youth, health, and perceived vitality – in sum, **her ability to successfully carry his children.**

Women's attraction, on the other hand, is more based on *psychology* – in particular, her assessment of a man's ability to care for her over time, and hence to successfully bring those children into adulthood. This assessment is a complex judgment that women make, consciously or not, with every man they meet. This is true regardless of whether she actually wants a baby – her response to men has been programmed into her over millions of years. Fundamentally, what determines a woman's psychological attraction to a man is her assessment of **his ability to care for her and her children.**

Now, this assessment has two components:

The first component is his perceived status – the wealth, power or influence, connections, or special skills that he has. Women are attracted to men who are more successful, popular or powerful than them. Women want men whom they believe will have something to offer them, who will increase their own status or security or quality of life.

The second component of a woman's psychological attraction comes from her assessment of whether a man is willing and able to focus that power to her benefit. This begins with her assessment of the quality of his attention on her and his responsiveness to her. Simply having power and influence is not enough. *The man must be willing and able to focus his power toward her, in a direction she likes, and in a sustained way.* This second component is the reason why talking to a woman about your power and wealth usually won't lead to sex. It does not indicate a willingness to take care of her, instead it highlights the amount of attention you have on yourself.

## Manson's key discovery: the importance of self-investment

 Manson made another important discovery – an encouraging one for men, because it provides a means of becoming immediately more attractive to women. ***Women are attracted to men whom they believe have the potential to become successful, as much as or more than they are attracted to men who are already successful.***

In other words, a man's potential future status is likely to be just as attractive to a woman as his current status – especially if he demonstrates the ability to give her quality attention and respond to her in the now. A high-status man who is emotionally unavailable or has no attention to give, is of no value to most women.

Manson's observation is good news for single men. The reason that your future success attracts her is that *she wants to go on the ride with you, the ride to your success. She wants to contribute to you*, which is another way of saying she wants to love you. The evolutionary force of love is working behind the scenes to get you dates – even if you spent the previous night on a park bench.

Manson's second breakthrough idea is this: A man demonstrates his potential to become successful by being *more invested in himself than he is in her or in the opinions of those around him.* He demonstrates this investment by how he relates to other people and how other people relate to him. ***This is the key to becoming an attractive man.*** If a man bends and waffles at every whim of his woman and everyone around him, if he lacks purpose and direction, if he is always agreeing with her out of laziness or lack of ideas, or if he is excessively hurt or incapacitated by rejection or disapproval, his success is doubtful, and therefore he becomes less attractive to her.

The important point here is that *"Investment in yourself"* is ultimately a matter of behavior and perception. And this is more good news for single men, because you can begin immediately to change your self-investment simply by how you behave – provided you do so authentically. You simply have to change your internal yardstick of success, your source of value and self-esteem, from external to internal measures. External measures could be whether she will go on a date with you or laugh at your jokes. Internal measures could be your felt-sense of connection with her, or your enjoyment (or not) of the interaction with her. **When you are not operating from an internal yardstick of success, she will feel it, and will become less attracted to you.**

*A man's excessive emotional investment in a woman, to the detriment of his investment in himself, is going to be a turn-off to her.* To the degree that you are too dependent on the opinion of others, and/or lacking a strong identity, purpose, and sense of self-worth, you will not be attractive to her. You will come across as emotionally unreliable, which reduces your value in her eyes. This is likely to be instinctual for her, not a conscious decision.

### Women's other attraction triggers: the source of her turn-on

What complicates the matter even further, and partially explains why so many men are so confused about female sexual attraction and clueless in creating it, is that women have several attraction triggers, in addition to the core one already discussed, which is her desire to be taken care of.

**Women get turned-on when they feel wanted,** or feel sexually attractive – typically as the result of men's expressed desire for them and their actions in pursuing them. This, of course, is a consequence of feminine sexual polarity: she is seeking to love in a feminine way, which is to attract and then magnify love, or give it back. Her core-feminine love-energy gets activated by feeling loved and wanted, and this manifests by her getting aroused.

*And this creates a big problem for men in the love and attraction game:* we want women to get turned on and to want us, and for this we must let them know, as directly as possible, that we want them. However, if we want them "too much", to the degree that we lack investment in ourselves, *it will turn them off.*

*This can feel, for men, like a game that they cannot win. But it's not.*

### The paradox of female sexual attraction – and the solution

The solution to this seeming paradox is quite simple – at least in theory – and it is to simultaneously do two things:

- First, let her know that you are attracted to her.

- Second, let her know that, as much as you are attracted to her, the actions that you take toward your success, self-esteem and self-concept do not depend on her acceptance or approval of you, or of anybody else.

*"Let her know"* doesn't necessarily mean to tell her directly either of these things. It is an attitude and way of being. Good communication however, direct or indirect, is the key to giving these two simultaneous messages: that you want her, but that you yourself are more important. This makes her feel secure in the fact that you are choosing her from a place of control and security in yourself, and not to fill some hole of validation.

According to Manson, the problem of almost all men who are attempting to engage women and not succeeding has to do with failure in their self-investment. It doesn't matter what you communicate around your self-investment. If you are not actually doing it, if it's not real, you will only get so far. Most women have an accurate "bullshit detector."

## "True confidence" vs. "salesmanship," and the problem of seduction techniques

Manson defines *"true confidence"* simply as a man's willingness to invest in himself. A man demonstrates this through his actions, his attitude, and his communications with the people around him. When it is authentic, a man's confidence is the greatest predictor of success in attracting quality women. When it is not authentic, it may generate *some* attraction – women can be somewhat gullible – but it always leads to problems. When confidence is not authentic, it *may* get you sex, but the quality of those relationships will not be satisfying, because you will be attracting women at a low level of development – your own level. Deep partnership with a woman requires a deep commitment to your own development. If your belief in yourself and commitment to your own development is low, you will attract partners who mirror that.

*Now, there is nothing wrong with attracting a partner at your level of development,* even if it's a low one. This is the function of relationship, and the value that women provide to men: they mirror our greatness, or lack thereof. We all play the games that we play, with the ultimate but often unconscious goal of becoming more loving, more fulfilled and more powerful human beings. As an intimacy advocate, I fundamentally believe that *any* intimacy is better than *no* intimacy. It all ends up in the same place eventually, which is an increase in our ability to love and to experience deep intimacy, sexual and not.

The problem, however, is that men are often disappointed by the number and/or quality of the partners they attract. *This may be because they are trying to compensate for an inherent lack of investment in themselves by becoming better salesmen.* They try and persuade women of the added value that they can bring. They try to impress them, rather than working to genuinely improve the "product," that is, themselves. They may become fabulous **pick-up artists** – they can get women turned-on, which can be of value to everybody, and they can try to make women believe that they have something valuable to offer. However, if the offer or the value is not authentic, if it's not coming from a true place of self-worth and of love, it will only attract women of a certain level of development and emotional maturity, and/or young and inexperienced women, women who do not yet know themselves and who will make you work really hard, and maybe pointlessly.

In other words, men avoid their own inner work, and instead try to develop techniques and short-cuts to get what they want, in this case women's love and sexual acceptance.

*Again – there is nothing wrong with techniques per se.* It's a core masculine strength to seek the quickest way to reach the goal. But short-cuts are not going to work if your goal is to play with the divine feminine in the field of sexual polarity. *You play with the divine feminine in women by "loving as best you understand love," by giving them all of the attention and acceptance that you have to give within the constraints of your need for self-investment and of your purpose, and finally by surrendering to them and taking their feedback as to how well you are doing.*

This is the **Man/Woman game**. It is likely to generate some fantastic sex, and by playing it well you may also be playing an important role in the transformation of global consciousness and the healing of the world.

### "Wanting her but not too much" becomes a false dichotomy

It's a false dichotomy because you can fully express your desire and attraction for a woman, thereby activating her feminine polarity to everyone's benefit – and yet still be highly invested in yourself.

*There is nothing wrong with letting her know how much you are attracted to her!* Indeed, to love her means to be authentic with her, at least to the degree that she wants you to be, and that includes letting her know how much you want her – *provided* that your desire for her is preceded and pre-empted by your investment in yourself. It's two parallel dimensions, not in opposition to each other, not at all.

Confusion over this apparent dichotomy is a big part of men's and women's suffering in relation to each other. It is one of the fundamental reasons that *"both halves of the human being, man and woman, have searched for each other for generations and always missed one another"* [Dieter Duhm].

We men might wish that women would have explained this to us earlier, that they would have helped us understand how they function in order to relate to them better. It would have been nice, and might have avoided a lot of grief, if our parents or first lovers had explained to us exactly what makes a woman become aroused, interested and attracted to us.

However, women themselves did not know this, or at least have failed to articulate it. They did not know it because **men and women can only fully know themselves in relation to the other.** Men and women have missed each other for generations. We are still searching for each other.

Women also could not articulate it because women are not the best resource for teaching men how to do our work, at least not through direct instruction. **Women want men to arouse them,** and they want men to invest in themselves because they love us and because it ultimately benefits them too. But women cannot lead or predict the direction of men's self-investment. That is the man's job.

## A long journey, but it's worthwhile

The work of investing in yourself will involve many aspects, including attitudes, actions and communications. These aspects will partly be related to things you do for yourself, and partly to how you communicate or demonstrate that self-investment to women, and how you relate to them from that place. *Investing deeply in yourself is really the only way to become an attractive man and to create deep partnerships with women.*

Some of these communications may be salesmanship, there is nothing wrong in that if the underlying product (you yourself) is solid. It is possible, for example, that the reason you are not attracting the women you want is because you have not yet figured out how to present your quality to the world, and hence are not creating resonance for the type of women you want to attract. You are perhaps insufficiently self-expressed, or too timid, or previous relationship failures have caused you to doubt yourself, and therefore you hold back.

However, the larger problem is that investing in yourself can be a long and arduous process. It can be a hard process that encompasses all aspects of your life. But it's a worthwhile journey. *"As a man, it may be the most worthwhile journey"* [Mark Manson].

Manson goes on to look at what *"self-investment"* actually means, in practice, and presents many additional and important attitudes and distinctions that are valuable when relating and communicating with women, and in playing the dating game.

But beyond the basic skills of self-investment, the following chapters will focus on four key skills:

- **The first skill is supporting and being of service to women by communicating with them in a way that fulfills their deep needs within their polarity.** If you start with true confidence, that is strong investment in yourself, if you have good attention on women and demonstrate your responsiveness to them, and if you then execute the emotional and physical communications described here, you will vastly increase the chances that she will become attracted to you. *"Having good attention"* means to increase the quality of your feeling-awareness, feedback, and appreciation. You can begin this process immediately. You can try to engage every feminine person you meet with the goal of becoming a more loving person, thus preparing you for that important encounter, and meanwhile transforming your relationships with all the women around you.

- **The second skill is to understand some key aspects of feminine people that are essential to know for relating powerfully to them.**

You will learn the secret reasons that feminine people behave the way they do, with effective ways to respond to them.

- *The third skill is to begin to understand female sexuality,* an area of vast misinformation for both sexes, and thereby begin to understand Sacred Sexuality. Sacred Sexuality, also known as "sex beyond ego-identification," is perhaps the most transformational thing that you will ever do. And it's free.

- *The fourth set of skills embodies some practical communication tools* and distinctions that could vastly deepen your partnerships with women and the quality of your emotional communication.

Onward...

# 12 Understanding and Executing the Feminine Commands

*"Give honest and sincere appreciation." – Dale Carnegie (Principle #2 of* How to Win Friends and Influence People*)*

*So, what do you actually do to play the Man/Woman game?* If you are primarily a masculine person and want to play a sexual polarity game with a woman – any woman, whether a friend or a date or a lover or a wife or colleague – this chapter will help you. If you are primarily a feminine person, read anyway as this chapter is a guide for practicing masculine love and will be applicable to many areas of your life.

As a prerequisite to success, you must be committed to *"love as best you understand love."* You execute this commitment by practicing the **Skills and Principles of Loving** as outlined Chapter 8. The first skill of loving is "Seeing," or paying attention. This is what you are going to be practicing, perhaps only for a minute or two, but perhaps for a lifetime.

Specifically, you will practice paying attention to women. Ideally, you will be committing to the happiness and well-being of all the women around you, whether you are attracted to them or not. If there is a specific woman or women that you care for and particularly want to practice with, that is good too. You might try and enlarge that small circle, however, since the more practice you can get, the more attractive you will become and the more quickly you will get results with that special woman... whether you already know her, or whether she is still in your future. It will also be more fun for you.

## So here is your mission

**With that in place, here is your Mission: to find women to whom you can communicate, directly or indirectly: "I want to support you and take care of you. Please help me to do this."**

You do not have to say this to her out loud. You merely have to demonstrate your support through your communications and actions. This is also known as loving her, caring for her, responding to her need, following her lead, accepting her direction, producing or providing for her, or accepting her command.

If you are actually able to say the words – *"I want to support you and take care of you"* – it can be very powerful. She may have never heard this from a man before, and it might really get her attention. She might not believe you, however, and so it may be better to just demonstrate your intention through your actions, and not to explicitly declare your intention.

Your support and caring for her can be for half a minute, as in opening a door for a woman, or a lifetime commitment. It doesn't matter because in that half-minute you will perform a miracle: *you will have loved a woman. You will be giving her your full attention for however long you decide you want to.* You will be with her fully and love her during that time.

You choose how much love you want to give her, and for how long. This is another reason why it might be best to just offer your support directly, rather than tell her what you are doing – in case you change your mind. You really only want to take care of her as long as it's fun or rewarding for you. However, if you *really* like her, and want to offer her unconditional support for a time, then you should definitely tell her directly. If she asks you why, tell her that you enjoy her company and would like an opportunity to get to know her and provide some value to her, no strings attached.

### Ways that you can support (or love) a woman

There are numerous ways that you can support and care for a woman. I am going to call this *"accepting her command"* – also known as responding to her need, or loving her. Assume that she will be continuously giving you commands, most of them non-verbal, most of the time that she is with you. Your job is to respond to these. Victor Baranco identified these transactions as **Call/Response.**

***The first way you can love her is to give her some practical help that she needs.*** Let's call this responding to an *"explicit command."* It could be an act of service, big or small, or a particular expertise that you have that she needs. Change a light bulb, fix her door handle, give her some information or a contact that will be helpful to her. Simply find out what she wants and then offer to do it.

If she makes a direct request for you to do something, or implies that it would please her if you would, then do it immediately – provided it fits your value system. *"Honey would you please take out the garbage... it would make me so happy!"* is an example of an excellent explicit command, as it will provide her a useful service, communicates the added value of that service (*"it will make me so happy"*), and will likely not contradict your value system.

> **"CALL/RESPONSE"**
>
> *This is the idea that men respond to women's "signals," sometimes consciously but often unconsciously. It is based on the notion that "Women call, men respond" – meaning that women are continuously putting out clues to what they want and to what would please them. Calling these clues "feminine commands" highlights the fact that women's signals must be received and responded to by men who hope to succeed with women.*

**The second way you can love her is to give her your attention and appreciation.** These *"implicit commands"* include *the art of paying attention, the arts of appreciation, validation, feedback and delight, and the art of complimenting.*

### Why respond to feminine "implicit commands"?

Well, simply because feminine people want these things whether they have asked for them or not. And they cost little or nothing for you to give. You can be proactive in your loving – she will love you for this and indeed this proactivity is one of the most adorable masculine traits for women. A woman wants you to be active and focused in your loving. Remember the feminine hunger: **what she wants is your awesome single-pointed consciousness and extraordinary masculine depth and discernment, focused on her and her goals. If you do this right, she will start feeling things for you and will want to play with you all day long. She will never get enough of you.**

You will find that fulfilling feminine implicit commands related to appreciation and validation is extraordinarily effective with feminine people. **Feminine people thrive on masculine attention and validation to a degree that masculine people can barely comprehend.** Of course, practice appreciation and validation with all people, men and women, but practice specifically with women, simply because they tend to be better receivers and will benefit more, which will empower you too.

I predict that once you start practicing these communication techniques, it will become a habit. You will never want to stop, and both your life and your bank account will be transformed, because you will have learned the greatest thing there is to learn: the art of human relationships [Dale Carnegie]. **You will likely have as many friends, lovers and money as you will ever want.**

A caveat: if you don't enjoy women being in love with you, are unwilling to commit that much outward attention, or can't handle that much affection directed towards you, you should not play this game. There are plenty of good games to play, you need not feel under any compulsion to play this one. Whether you like to play hard with women like I do, or prefer a more gentle style, please do believe that there is at least one woman waiting for you who wants to play the exact game that you do. Start with the Skills and Principles of Loving, and improvise from there. Take what you like and leave the rest. You will not go wrong.

### Some practical examples of supporting and caring for a woman

Supporting a woman and paying attention to her can be infinitely varied, and very entertaining. Let's start with the basics. The prime directive is: **pay attention, listen, and reflect back.** If you need to get her engaged in conversation first, see Chapter 16. For the rest, it could take any number of forms, including:

- Look her in the eye and smile.

- Ask leading questions. These are questions that bring out her thoughts, feelings, and dreams. Invite her to talk. However, if you find her boring, or even repelling, you will need to either move on or try something new.

- Maintain an attitude of interested and delighted attention.

- Feedback what you see of her internal state: *"You look happy/sad/ upset talking about this,"* and also take guesses: *"Did you feel angry when that happened?"*

- Feedback your reactions to her in a way that validates her experience: *"That must have been hard," "I felt happy/sad when you said that."* Amplify your response when you are genuinely moved by her, or attracted to something she said or how she is being. ***This is important. Get excited for her, she will love it.***

- Confirm to her as frequently as possible your interest and attention on her: *"I hear you," "I am with you," "I am listening," "this is the most interesting conversation / nicest thing anyone has said to me all day," "you are making my day," "I love talking to you."*

- Thank her and appreciate her for sharing her thoughts and feelings with you: *"I love that you trust me enough to tell me these things,"* or just *"Thank you for saying that."* Always end any conversation or interaction with a woman with an appreciation: *"I enjoyed so much talking to you – I find you very interesting and cool," "you have such a beautiful smile," "you look like a fun person,"* or even *"that went well didn't it?"*

- Align with everything she says as much as you can. Treat this as an inviolate rule, and get creative. Never lie to her, of course, instead find a way to align, if at all possible. At minimum, acknowledge her right to her opinion. Say it and mean it: *"I honor your right to think and feel as you do,"* or (when you can't stand how she is being) *"I am sure there is a good reason that you are being this way."* This is especially important when she is giving you negative feedback. You may need to assert yourself. You can try to do this nicely and without putting her down or making her wrong – though it's not always easy.

- Give her gifts, open car doors, fetch things for her, drive her places, run errands, research and organize fun events for her, walk on the street-side... the full range of chivalrous gestures. It will be fun for her and you both.

- Compliment her for her clothing, jewelry, appearance, poise, intelligence, sense of humor, generosity, attention, kindness, resourcefulness, energy... really anything you notice yourself liking about her.

- Be well-dressed and well-groomed all the time. This is an implicit compliment to a feminine person – it demonstrates that you want to please her.

- If you see her responding, you can amplify by flirting with her and touching her. This is such an important topic it is covered in Chapter 17.

- Be guided by your own instincts. As you become proficient you may find yourself responding in your gut to a woman's energy field. Anything that you can do or say to a woman that makes her look more alive or that puts a smile on her face is furthering your goal of loving her. You will feel her in your body and you can be guided by that – even if she says nothing.

Fundamentally, you are trying to *increase the quality of your attention and feeling-awareness, and then communicate from that place.* You are simply connecting your eyes and ears (observation) to your brain and mouth (expression). This is a creative process that will require you be in tune with her unspoken emotions and needs; and also with yourself, your needs, and your emotional and physical response to her. And unfortunately, there is no short-cut to learning how to do this. Everyone is still learning, always. But you must begin.

### How honest and direct can you be?

Probably much more honest and direct than you can even imagine. Many of us have an intense and irrational fear of approaching strangers with any kind of real emotion or need, which is even culturally drummed into us as inappropriate; but the truth is that most people are looking for authentic emotional connection, even when they don't immediately respond to it or even admit it. If you think that what I am describing sounds like it might be extremely difficult and uncomfortable, particularly with strangers, then think again. You are probably aiming too small. These kinds of conversations happen all the time, and even between strangers. But it all begins with the simple practices of *paying attention and acknowledging / appreciating.* If all you do is that, you will be golden.

If you are in a marriage or a relationship that has gone flat and you don't even know where to begin to rekindle the flame, or if you are single and the thought of talking to a strange woman causes your knees to shake and your mind to go blank, just do one thing: *notice something you like and approve about her, no matter how small, and let her know.* Then see how she responds.

If she responds negatively, acknowledge that and apologize: *"I am sorry,*

*I hope it did not offend you that I said that,"* or *"sorry that did not quite come out as I intended,"* or even *"that was dumb, wasn't it."* However she responds, align with her – even if she is behaving like a bitch (from your perspective).* There is a good reason that she is being like this. ***Honor her right to think and feel as she does.***

Most of the time, however, she will respond positively. More than likely she will smile at you and brighten visibly. She will start to become interested in you. When that happens, smile back and notice something else about her that you approve of or find interesting. It could be almost anything. Perhaps not a body part, at least with a stranger, but jewelry or clothing is perfect, the contents of her shopping cart, something she is doing, how she is being or an energy about her, how she talks. ***And then keep on going as long as you can or until it stops being fun.***

If she looks like she is done with you, appreciate her and move on. You can even leave her with a compliment for rejecting you: *"You look like a woman who knows her mind / is on a mission."* If you know her already (maybe she is your wife), and you really can't think of anything else to say or do for her, try asking her directly: *"What could I do right now that would put a smile on your face,"* or even the most direct: *"How can I serve you now, what would you like from me, what would you like to hear from me now?"* ***Directness and curiosity are among the greatest gifts you can give a feminine person.***

To summarize: let her know, verbally or non-verbally, that she has your full attention. Then wait for her command (her call or signal), and failing that simply do the things that you know work with feminine people. And fine-tune that based on her response. In a worst-case scenario, when you are not picking up any signal at all, ***start with interested and delighted attention and you likely won't go wrong.***

It's that simple. Anyone can do it. All it takes is a little attention, willingness, and some courage. You may not be a genius at this right away, but it won't be long before you get some responses or feedback that will blow your mind. And very soon, you will be a lot closer to a woman than you were before, and you will be visibly having a good time, which will make you more attractive and interesting.

You can use these techniques with a new woman or with your current partner – the effect will be identical. Remember the single greatest cause of failed relationship: ***We are lazy and stingy with our love.*** We don't say the things that we care for and appreciate about other people. *Don't make that mistake!* Do not withhold your approval of her or your attraction to her. Do your masculine duty and lead in communication. Set the tone of the relationship by being willing to listen to her and put your attention on her. Give back the lead when she wants it, but you go first. *"Men first in danger, women first in pleasure"* [Victor Baranco].

# 13 The Importance of Authenticity

*"Providing quality information to the men in your life will help your man succeed by making you happy, which is exactly the outcome he's hoping for" – Alison Armstrong*

To be successful in this game, there is one additional requirement: *you must respond to her authentically and communicate your true thoughts and feelings.* "Communicating your true feelings" does not mean communicating all your feelings to her all the time *("You are beautiful to me and I want to fuck you"* – although there may be a place for that too). It means communicating as much as you think she wants to hear. But everything you say to her must be as truthful as you know how.

Early on, as you witness the extraordinary impact of these techniques, you may wonder if you are being authentic with her or just giving her a line. You may even go wild, pushing the limits of the type of compliments and appreciation that you are able to give, or that you have the courage to say out loud. This mainly indicates that you are working hard at this. Remember, you need only "love as best you understand love," and it is not a crime to say something to a woman in the hope of pleasing her that comes out totally dumb-ass. If it lands badly, apologize, even if you don't know what you did wrong. If it lands well, but you are not sure it was totally authentic, her response to you might make it authentic.

For example: a woman to whom you say, *"You look beautiful today,"* may become beautiful to you. Simply use your best discernment, realizing that sometimes you just have to hear the words out of your mouth before you can know if they really fit. Women are the same, actually, if not worse, so they can't blame you. You will often be able to correct yourself after speaking: *"Actually that was not entirely accurate,"* or *"Let me qualify that."* You will sometimes come out with a real doozer, and this is fine because your next utterance will be a more loving or more engaging expression. Don't knock yourself. Just *"love as best you understand love."*

It doesn't have to be a big deal either. A smile or a kind word can go a very long way. You might, in five seconds, make a person's day.

Remember: **_Feminine people love, more than anything else, to be seen and appreciated._** If you learn to do this well, you will have a spectacular life.

## What if you really think she is behaving abominably?

You will need to get creative. It is possible, in almost every situation, to find an authentic empathic response. You can try saying nothing while sending her love and empathy non-verbally[7]. You can also revert back to _"I am sure there is a good reason you are being like this"_ or _"you have a right to feel the way you do,"_ or _"I think I see your point."_ These can be true statements coming from a higher perspective, but if you can't _feel_ the truth of them, or say them _authentically_, then don't. Say nothing, or just walk away. We return to this topic in the next chapter.

But whatever you do, do not say something that you know upfront is insincere or inauthentic, just to get her attention, or even her body, or to shut her up or shut her down. That would not be playing this game correctly. And you will be damaging the efforts of all the men who will follow in your footsteps. **_It is unkind and irresponsible to do this, and a crime towards your brothers, all of us who love women, who will need to work harder with her next time because you have betrayed her._**

---

7    Try a practice called HeartMath, heartmath.com, or use NVC (Chapter 36)

# 14 Responding to Negative Feedback from a Woman

*"Don't just do something, be there."* – *Marshall Rosenberg*

*"When we are angry, killing people is too superficial."* – *Marshall Rosenberg*

It can be painful for a man to receive negative feedback, or even outright rejection from a woman. But there is a positive way to think about it. When a woman gives you negative feedback, she is telling you what you are doing that stands in the way of loving her, and she is giving you information on how you can please her and love her better next time. She is giving you a great gift. Absolutely commit to thoughtfully and gracefully receiving all negative feedback from feminine people: find her right and align with her, as much as possible. Acknowledge internally her right to let you know how she feels. You can do even better, if possible, and *thank her* for letting you know how she feels. **She is giving you the opportunity to learn about her and about yourself, and to use that information to become more loving towards everyone.**

Always, as much as possible but *"within your value system,"* encourage and support a woman to share her feelings with you. Women may have a lot of fear and anger about asking for what they want and need, and about sharing negative feelings. They will often express themselves with a lot of defensiveness, resentment, shame and blame. Do not take this personally. Instead, listen for the hidden message, the needs underlying all her communications, and understand that she may have a lifetime of previous upset around these issues, making it difficult for her to express herself clearly and cleanly.

*This is, actually, one of the most impactful things you can ever do with a feminine person.* If you actively encourage her self-expression, even when it is negative feedback for you, she may be absolutely floored. She may have never received this from a man before. She may be stunned into silence, begin to wonder where you came from, and start looking at you like a God. You may change her life in one moment, and she may remember you for the rest of her days. You will wonder why you waited so long to do something like this, and kick yourself for all your previous years of arguing with women.

Remember also that for thousands of years women have been oppressed, raped and sometimes killed for expressing independent thought and feeling, so this is going to be a much bigger deal for her than it is for you. Bite your tongue and say nothing more than *"yes thank you"* or *"yes ma'am,"* or even just *"got it."* It will cost you just a little, but it may be huge for her.

Sometimes you may feel that you need to argue with negative feedback, or present your alternate viewpoint. That is just fine, but first do the following. Thank her and appreciate her for sharing with you. Reassure her of your deep desire to know *all her feelings,* and especially the negative ones. Make sure she is done: *"Thank you – is there more?"* Give it a good moment of silence while gazing at her adoringly. And finally, respond humbly and with her permission: *"Would you mind if I suggested another point of view? Would you be willing to hear my response to this?"*

### The fundamental reason why taking negative feedback is difficult

Receiving negative feedback is difficult for everyone. In fact, women are often no better at it than men. *Almost everyone goes wrong here, at least initially.* For many people, rejecting feedback becomes a chronic attitude that blocks deeper forms of relationship and limits the depth of intimacy with our partners, or even any serious friendship or business collaboration. When you encounter these extreme cases, you may have no option but to move on.

There are ways to give negative feedback that are easier to hear and more likely to be successful. The most important of these are Marshall Rosenberg's Non-Violent Communication (NVC, see Chapter 36), the practice of Withholds (Chapter 37) and *"You don't need to get what you want if you can express what you want"* (Chapter 40). The latter two are the necessary preparation for giving negative feedback – clearing out your own **Emotional Charge** so that you can communicate more effectively. You can, and should, definitely use NVC, or whatever works for you, when you are giving negative feedback.

However, when receiving negative feedback, you may have no choice. Interrupting someone who is giving you negative feedback in order to request that they use NVC, or try and educate them on how you want to be talked to, is not generally a good strategy. Maybe afterwards, when they are done and have calmed down and feel heard. It is always difficult to respond lovingly to a communication expressed as a judgment or a demand, or that is delivered with a lot of anger. But you can try. You can listen for the feelings and needs underlying all human communications, even those communications that are expressed as judgments or demands, and respond to them from that place. **This is a primary aspect of leading in communication.** You model, or demonstrate, the behavior and the style of communication, and of listening, that you are seeking from the other. You discern their deeper feelings and needs, whether they have stated them or not, and then mirror them back. This is much more effective than telling them how you want them to talk to you. It is the loving thing to do. *It is, in fact, one of the highest forms of love.*

*"Modeling listening skills"* doesn't mean that you become a doormat. You can assert, but always lovingly. You must learn to **not make her wrong** and you do this by *learning to speak in the language of feelings and needs* [Marshall Rosenberg]. They cannot effectively argue with you from a statement of your feelings and needs – if they try, you just repeat yourself. Speaking in this way is difficult. It requires,

> ### EMOTIONAL CHARGE
>
> *"Emotional charge" is in the nature of raw, unprocessed emotion. It is when we are triggered by something that happens, and have a gut reaction, but don't fully know why. We feel, perhaps, that our response is disproportionate to the triggering event. The problem with emotional charge is that it blocks effective communication, as the other person senses our charge and responds to that, the unspoken emotion, rather than our words. We return to this problem and explain how to deal with it in Chapter 37: Withholds*

in many cases, a complete re-wiring of our communication patterns, of our listening and speaking. However, it is possible, and extraordinarily effective.

To receive negative feedback more gracefully, it may help to ask ourselves why it is so difficult, and why so many people simply reject it outright. Perhaps we do this out of pride or ego, but **most people who compulsively reject feedback, do so out of low self-esteem and self-doubt originating from internalized oppression.** We don't feel we can take it, we imagine it would kill us, we can't stand to hear other people truth about us. Maybe we lack the internal strength to *"take what you like and leave the rest"* [Alcoholics Anonymous] and so we reject it all, or don't even hear it. *"Lack of internal strength" is the same as low self-esteem.* When you realize that someone is rejecting your feedback out of low self-esteem, it could give you more empathy for them, which will help you make a better communication. When you realize that you yourself may be rejecting feedback out of low self-esteem, you may be humbled by this awareness, but you will grow from it.

To grow in relationships, we must truly *respond to the other.* Without response, there is no relationship, and without relationship there is no manifestation. You may as well be alone.

## Negative feedback is always useful

The reason negative feedback is always useful, is that it almost always reveals a dimension of the truth. Let me prove this to you. Suppose someone calls you a broccoli, or a grape. You would probably laugh and ask them what they mean. Now imagine someone close to you calls you selfish, immature, and arrogant. Would you be more upset than in the first scenario? Most probably yes, because you would sense an element of truth. Even if it were not the *whole truth*, it is highly likely that you have moments of selfishness, immaturity and arrogance. This core truth is the fundamental reason that the truest and most helpful response to negative feedback is almost always to say "thank you".

There may be times when you don't relate at all to somebody's feedback. You may, in fact, be completely convinced that it is entirely their own projection and has nothing to do with you. You might be tempted to argue with them. But try and resist that temptation. If you must, tell them gently that you are not sure that you relate to what they are saying, but that you will certainly think about it. Even if their accusation is not true in that moment, there will likely come a time, a day or a month or a year later, that you catch yourself starting to behave in the way that they have described to you – and you will remember that thing they said, and stop yourself. Maybe you will avoid making a costly mistake, and you will be grateful to that person. So, short-cut that delay and be grateful to them now instead.

***Here is the gift of negative feedback: even when it's "off" (inaccurate) it will almost always push you in the direction that you ought to be going in anyway.*** For instance: somebody gives you negative feedback about a project or a person that you are about to engage, as a consequence of which you still choose to engage, but do so with more caution and more discernment.

Let me say it again: learning to accept negative feedback is one of the most important and effective practices for learning how to love and for becoming more inter-related. Wise men and women do even more than accept negative feedback – they actively seek it out. *The day that you start actively seeking out negative feedback, is the day that you will achieve true personal power.*

## When you need to walk away

You can choose, if you wish, to be present and empathic to a person who is speaking to you in an angry, repetitive way and is not listening, even after repeated attempts of yours to assert yourself. Or you can choose to walk away. Both options are acceptable. Walking away, however, may be seen as an aggressive act, and is therefore a measure of last resort. Some situations call for it. Indeed, in some situations any other response than walking away might be inauthentic, a violation of healthy boundaries, or even dangerous to you.

In a later chapter we will explain the concept of **giving within your surplus.** This is the same as *"loving within your value system".* It means that there is a limit to your kindness, generosity, and empathy. You can push those boundaries, but you must not go beyond your ability to respond authentically to people. You will know you have gone beyond your surplus because you will feel angry and resentful afterwards, or simply upset without fully knowing why. It is not helpful in relationship to do this. You are actually betraying both yourself and the other person, who may sense your resistance and will not be gratified by you, or grow from the interaction. You will have given your time and attention, and just created even more upset. Not all problems are yours to solve.

People go beyond their surplus typically because they try and behave in a way that they think they should, or they have been told they should. It is an inauthentic response, and they pay the price for it afterwards, and feel distant from the person they are trying to help. This does not help anyone. Women are particularly prone to this, due to their socialization, and need to be very vigilant in this area. We return to this topic in Chapter 29 on women's over-pleasing.

# 15 What You Should N*ever* Say to a Woman

Whatever you do, *do not ever, ever tell a woman how to think or feel.* For two reasons.

The first reason is that your telling a woman how she should feel is simply ludicrous. It is tantamount to a gorilla telling you how to program a computer. *A masculine person cannot possibly understand the feminine range of feelings and processing style.* The very best you can do is be willing for her to teach you. This in itself is enough for a lifetime. You must be humble. She will make you work, but it's the finest work that you will ever do: helping a woman to heal is healing the world. A happy woman is an extraordinarily powerful being. You may have released a woman to her full potential and reason for being (which is her love), and if so you may have *"fired a shot that is heard around the world"* [Werner Erhard, quoting Ralph Waldo Emerson ]. You have no idea – no idea – how much good she may do after you have helped her heal herself. But you can bet your last dollar that you and all men and women everywhere will benefit.

The second reason for not telling a woman how to think and feel is this*: she will want to kill you.* It will destroy any chances you have of making a difference to her. So stay clear. If you screw up, beg her forgiveness. Women are easily upset, at least from men's perspective, but they also (usually) forgive easily. Especially when they feel a man's sincere remorse and adoration.

# 16 Initiating and Maintaining a Conversation

*"You miss 100% of the shots that you don't take."* – Wayne Gretzky

Initiating a conversation with a new woman (say in a public place or at an event) is not that difficult. As in any communication it will challenge your creativity, but that is to be expected.

When you want to initiate a conversation with a new woman, you would apply the same communication skills as you would with someone you know. Actually it makes no difference that she is a stranger to you, because that condition only lasts a moment anyway.

When you start playing this game, it may be difficult to gather up the courage to say something flirtatious to a strange woman. But as you practice, it will come easier and easier to you.

Many men are terrified of talking to an attractive woman. If you have already mastered this, I take off my hat to you – you are ahead of the game, so now you can take it to the next level and try loving her. But even if you are afraid of talking to strange attractive women, and in answer to the never-ending quest for good opening lines, here are some honest approaches that have worked for me:

*The best place to meet women is somewhere you have a common interest.* If you don't like bars, do not try and pick up women in bars. Supermarkets are OK, everyone goes food shopping and you are therefore guaranteed to find a representative sample of womankind in a grocery store. Actually, a surprising number of meetings happen in grocery stores, especially health-food stores. You have to be there anyway, so you may as well make the best of it and have as much fun as you can. But even better is a hiking club, church, music or theater event, painting class, restaurant meet-up, or any place of mutual interest. Events give you an immediate opener, because you have something in common besides a random encounter: ask her what she thinks of the event. If she responds to you, you are off to the races. You may have an extremely interesting conversation with her. You can take some risks in self-disclosure here too. Just remember to be interested and to ask leading questions.

*Say the first thing that pops into your head.* Don't hesitate, don't over-think. Your communication will be 80% non-verbal anyway, so what you actually say doesn't matter as much as you might imagine. *"Say, that's a great-looking cabbage in your shopping cart – tell me, please how do you cook it?"* That is a simple example of a good opener because you are:

- Noticing something about her;

- Asking her a leading question with a high probability she has a ready answer;

- Leveraging the humble cabbage toward a potential common interest (in cooking).

Everything you say initially to a strange woman should end with a question. You can even open flat-out with a question, with no preambles, once you have made eye contact with her: *"Do you like this store?"* Take a chance. The worst that can happen is that she will say *"yeah"* and look bored, at which point you can either smile sweetly, or tell her your favorite thing about this store and ask what she likes. Most women have more tolerance for stupid questions than you may imagine. And particularly when they sense *men's interested and delighted attention on them, and our desire to get to know them.*

**Your flirts will be more successful if your internal condition is a happy and confident place.** From that state of mind, you will easily see good opportunities, you may be surprised at how many present themselves to you. Don't over-think, don't worry about whether you are going to get anywhere with her, such as giving her your card or asking for her number so you can call her. Focus on your moment with her, and the feeling of triumph you will feel after you have successfully engaged a woman who is attractive to you, and/or have put a smile on the face of a woman you are not necessarily attracted to. And take that energy into your next encounter. Every positive experience, no matter how minuscule, increases your readiness for that important encounter, which brings it to you sooner.

Here is another great secret of men who are successful at meeting women: **Increase the flow of people through your life.** You have to get out of the house and go to events where the type of woman you want to meet is going to hang out. You can also leverage your network – tell all your friends (especially women friends) that you want to meet someone, and try and describe to them what you are looking for. This idea is from Susan Page's excellent book, **IF I AM SO WONDERFUL WHY AM I STILL SINGLE?**

***Golden Rule: it is much better to be "interested" than "interesting."*** If you go to a party and have the intention only of listening to people and getting to know them, you will be absolutely amazed at how many people will describe you as a great conversationalist.

A caution: In places that are traditionally considered women's territory such as yoga and dance classes, your flirting may not be well received. The authentic approach is to be there for the activity itself, and demonstrate that by continuing to attend. It's possible that she will be more receptive to you after she has seen you a few times. It also creates a great opener, *"Hey I saw you here yesterday! Isn't this a great class?"* You noticed and remembered her, and you share an enthusiasm. It's also possible that she has no interest in men at this point in her life, in which case you can give yourself kudos both for doing something good for yourself (attending a great class) and reaching out to a woman you are attracted to. Not all your days will be so good.

In case you are rejected, do not, under any circumstances show anger or upset. It may create a most unpleasant situation, which will be far worse for you than it is for her. Since you are the evil aggressor and you are persisting in your attitude, she may gather all her friends to defend her... and shun you. If you have the courage to smile and thank her (verbally or non-verbally) for setting boundaries with you, do it. Apologize gracefully if you can and if it would not make the situation worse. Say: *"I get it. I am very sorry if I was inappropriate and made you uncomfortable."* By simply apologizing for the fact that you might have occurred to her as inappropriate, and expressing genuine remorse for any hurt or discomfort you may have caused, ***you are accepting her right to think and feel as she does.*** If you are able to say those words sincerely, her mouth is likely to drop and she will stare at you in disbelief. This unusual experience might forever change how she relates to men.

***Likewise, and whatever else you do, never defend yourself.*** There is no need. You are a man and you love women. You may want to work toward having no problem at all being corrected by women. Eventually you might even learn to enjoy it: it indicates that you are a winner.

You will likely find these techniques quite easy to apply once you stop over-thinking. If you should falter and lose hope on the obstacle course towards intimacy that women and society place in men's way, just remind yourself: *you are on a mission from the Goddess.* You are here to serve womankind in general, and specifically the woman (or women) who will eventually approve of you and accept you. You cannot fail in your mission because it is divinely inspired. If you want to cry, go find a brother and wail on his shoulder for a while. And then throw yourself back into the fray. Even better, enroll your brother in storming your next yoga class. It's more fun with a friend. It's also more effective: it is social proof that you are not a serial killer, since you have at least one friend. Everybody knows that serial killers don't run in pairs.

## What if she is boring you — or even repelling you?

This is a tricky situation. To let a woman ramble on as you get increasingly bored and uncomfortable is not a loving thing to do. If it's just for a little bit, you can enjoy her essence, her intention, and the fact that she is reaching out to you even if you don't find her interesting and/or are not attracted to her. If you stretch yourself you might find that you actually do get interested. But don't go beyond your threshold.

You can always walk away (ideally with a compliment), or you can try and change the conversation. You have to do it without making her wrong or saying directly that she is boring you, but it's almost always possible. Finding something interesting about someone is actually one of the core skills of loving (and also in the art of being a good conversationalist).

So, follow the Golden Rule: **be interested in her and acknowledge her for something she is saying or doing.** Let's say, for example, she is going on about some concert she went to, and you really don't care. You might say, *"It sounds like a great experience,"* or *"I get that you really love the music,"* and then make the switch: *"…but I am actually most curious about ___. What do you think about ___?"*

Or you can be even more direct and ask for the attention back on yourself. Asking a woman for advice is an almost certain win. *"Wow, thanks for sharing all that about ___, but I wanted to ask you some advice about / your opinion about…."* Or even (maybe you are trying to tell a story and she is interrupting you): *"You know I would love to finish my story, because I would like to hear your thoughts about it afterwards."* Or else just smile and interrupt her with a bold compliment: *"You are so animated talking about this! That is so charming!"*

The definition of a successful interaction with a woman is not one that is filled with chatter, but one where you feel a connection. If you feel it in your body, she will likely feel it too. She will wonder what happened, and you will know: *you gave her your full attention.* She may not be accustomed to this. And she may be intrigued.

# 17 Complimenting and Flirting

*"To a large extent, 'free love' consists in giving and positive offensive."*
*– Dieter Duhm*

In addition to drawing out a woman's ideas and feelings and letting her know you are interested in her, you will want to compliment and flirt with her if you think she will be at all responsive, and so long as it's not totally inappropriate.

It's not necessarily about dating her, it's about putting a smile on her face and making her giggle. It doesn't matter whether or not you are sexually attracted to her. In fact, flirting with people you may not be sexually attracted to is hugely satisfying. If you are single and looking, here is a practice I most strongly recommend to you: flirt with any woman, of any age, who crosses your field of vision and whom you imagine might enjoy it. You will not be single very long, simply because you will be having so much fun it will draw people to you.

## So what is a flirt?

Essentially it's an amplified appreciation that includes a clear though subtle sexual suggestion. It is the sexual suggestion that makes the flirt powerful but also delicate. You should only flirt with a woman who wants it, and at a time that works for her. You may, therefore, want to begin with a small flirt to test her receptivity.

Compliments and flirting are extremely effective with almost all feminine people and particularly when starting a relationship. Give as many compliments as you can think of on a date, more is always better. If you do nothing but appreciate and validate her you are almost certain to make a difference to her. But compliments with flirts might take things over-the-top, you might make her day and you may eventually also get her in bed, if such is your mutual desire.

Compliments or flirts can either be outrageous or quietly sincere and heartfelt. You will need to experiment to find your particular style. One of my personal favorites is, *"You are so clever and so beautiful."* This works for me because I truly value both of those qualities (remember that compliments must be authentic, the same as anything else you say to a woman). *"You are very funny,"* or *"how did you get so funny"* are also popular. *"You know you want it"* can be good, depending on the state of the relationship. *"I want you"* can be fun as well. This is not exactly a compliment, but your desire for her is an implicit compliment. Use your imagination and the perfect compliment will jump out at you. And when that happens, do not hesitate. Say it immediately or your fear will get the best of you.

Your sincere or authentic compliment will be effective in proportion to the extent that the woman has not yet fully acknowledged herself, or feels secure in that area. For example: saying *"you look beautiful today"* to a classically beautiful woman is good – if you mean it and have no ulterior motive besides pleasing her. But saying the same thing to a woman who may not know she is attractive may get you a home run

Don't be afraid of going over the top on compliments. At worst she will challenge you and resist the compliment, but it can be entertaining to argue the sincerity of a compliment with the recipient. You actually can't lose on this one – the more she argues the more you come back with your sincerity. You can even amplify your compliments and make a game of making her blush to the roots of her hair. She wants to be convinced of your sincerity and is therefore on your side, regardless of what she says.

## The ethics of flirting

When is it wrong to flirt with a woman?

Well first and foremost, when she doesn't want it. She will let you know. You will likely feel it in your body ("oops…"). If that happens, no need to explain or apologize. Just stop immediately. You can continue your positive appreciations – unless you have lost her completely, but that will be rare. Just tone it down.

The second reason to stop flirting is if she is over-responding to you and you are certain you are not physically attracted to her, or interested in her company. Remember, you are trying to put a smile on her face, not to mess with her head. *Golden Rule: if she is smiling at you and you are enjoying yourself, you are likely doing well.* But use your judgment and stay tuned to your insides, your felt-awareness of yourself and of her.

# 18 Escalation: You Have Rapport. Or Not.

*"Most people are very diligent in their daily struggle against sexuality... Sometime or another, we have all fought a heroic battle against our desires, and we have been defeated by them." – Dieter Duhm*

Once you see a woman responding to you, you have three choices. You can:

- Continue what you are doing and amplify it (take more risks or become more outrageous in your appreciation);

- Make a request;

- End the conversation.

Your request can be anything: ask her out on a date, or tell her you must go now but would she like to continue the conversation later. Ask her anything that you would want from her, anything at all. Be direct and to the point and ideally accompany it with a feeling statement: *"You are such an interesting person, would you be willing to ___?"* You can be completely outrageous in your request, if you dare: *"I am shy to ask you this as I don't normally pick-up women in supermarkets, but I'd like to see you again,"* or even the most direct: *"I enjoy speaking with you, may I see you again?"*

If you wish to end the conversation with no further action, simply tell her you have enjoyed speaking with her and walk away. You can also double your impact, if you wish, by leaving her with a compliment or a flirt.

## What if she is *not* responding to you  (or worse – you piss her off)?

If a woman is not responding to you after several attempts, end the conversation or abort your approach. The fact that you are committed to loving women doesn't mean you have to kill yourself working for them. If she's not doing her part, walk away. She doesn't fancy you, at least not today – you can try again tomorrow. Cool your heels, and thank her internally for not wasting your time. Look for another woman who is more responsive to you. She likely won't be far away.

If you get clobbered in the interaction and start feeling angry, discouraged or depressed, take a break from your mission. Find a brother and cry on his shoulder, this is what brothers are for. You will empower him too by asking him for what you need – don't be afraid to practice directness with men too. Do something nice for yourself – pick up the phone and call a friend, go to the gym, lose yourself in some project or in computer games. Do some reflection or self-forgiveness, o whatever you need to do to return to the game as soon as possible, bold refreshed and renewed.

# 19 The Fundamental Problem of Women

*"None of us wants to grow up." – Cheri Huber*

If everything I have been talking about in this section occurs to you as just some silly game (or worse, contrived, insincere or a con-job), and you can't put your heart into it – then don't play. This is the fastest game I know to play with feminine people and will likely get you spectacular results on all important measures, but you *will* cause some upset in others. You will also be challenging your own internal limitations, particularly at the level of your self-confidence, perception, self-awareness and feeling-awareness, use of language, and reactivity. *If you are not willing to risk causing upset in others, or to challenge your internal limitations, don't play this game.*

It's also very likely that some people, men or women, won't like the game. They may even challenge the notion of a "game" when relating to other people. Or else they might say *"Just come from the heart"* or *"get out of your head"* – which is not bad advice, of course you should do that, but this kind of advice implies that loving people is incompatible with an active process of feeling-awareness, communication, and appreciation. They may want to be loved in a different way, or they may critique your style. Maybe they don't agree that *"love is an intention,"* or else they have the very common belief that love just happens, and that a conscious intention to increase it kills it or depletes its value.

People have all kinds of needs and they may just not fit in to what you are doing, or resonate with you. Of course you can listen to their feedback and take it in, indeed taking negative feedback to heart is very important in this game. *But don't stop playing.* Be aware too that there are all kinds of ways to do relationships and the fact that somebody doesn't like your game doesn't make either you or them wrong. *"In relationship, everyone is right,"* but you still need to realize that this is a powerful game, possibly *the* most powerful game you can play with feminine people, and you *will* get resistance.

Resistance to genuine appreciation, emotional connection and dating can come from any number of sources, but here is a major one. Many women have all kinds of ideas of what they want from a masculine partner, some of which could be completely unrealistic or purely a consequence of social conditioning – not what they deeply want at all, not the thing that would transform them irrevocably. Most people have deep social conditioning and hang-ups around man/woman relationships and sexuality. This is sad because the result is that we miss out on one of the greatest things that life has to offer: true sexual intimacy and deep partnership, the most profound and most fulfilling of human experiences.

Wise men know that they can never fully understand women, but many women imagine that they can understand men. They think that if men behaved more like women, if men did the things that women naturally do and without being asked, then everyone would be happier. They imagine that men can be fixed, or that they could find a masculine partner who would be capable of proactively sensing and responding to their needs in the way a woman can, or who could feel and communicate like women do. This is unlikely to happen. Men are not *"misbehaving women"* [Alison Armstrong]. There is a good reason that men are the way they are.

## The fundamental problem of women

*The fundamental problem of both women and men, with regards to the way they relate to each other, is that they are uneducated and lazy, or stingy.* Many women are hurt and angry, and deeply mistrust men, perhaps due to multiple previous betrayals. They have a right to feel this way, and yet they will need to get over it if they want to heal themselves and find their true power. You can help them, up to a point, by listening to them and providing empathy, by attempting to enter their world, by becoming more *trustable*; but ultimately they need to forgive and let go. *"None of us wants to grow up"* [Cheri Huber[8]]. "Growing up" means finding and expressing our true individuality, and loving well. Loving well means managing our emotional life in order to create our own happiness, which includes relating to people from where they are at, not from where we would like them to be. This is the fundamental human growth challenge and it applies to both men and women. Many women are not yet ready to relate to men from where they are at.

---

8   See "There is Nothing Wrong with You" by Cheri Huber. Huber is the founder and guiding teacher of the Zen Monastery Peace Center located in Murphys, California. The center runs week-long retreats focused on meditation and psychodrama, which are designed to give you self-awareness around the multitude of internal voices that constantly tell you that there is, actually, something wrong with you.

*As a consequence of all this, through a combination of past hurts and betrayals, and their own laziness and lack of education about men and how men operate, women often feel angry and alone.* This may be true whether they are single, or else in a relationship or marriage that has gone flat – or worse. Either situation will make them angry if their deep needs are not being met. But many are not willing to do their part. You can help them to see this, if you first find them right, or accept them, in the place where they are. You can give them your attention, your love and approval, which is what they really want; but sometimes their opening response will be to dump on you all of the accumulated negative feelings they have towards the clueless men who preceded you, and towards a society that puts them down and constantly invalidates them. You can only accept this, empathize with them as best you can, while staying within your value system – that is, be direct, and do not push your empathy beyond what you have to give.

Women can play their side of this game and heal themselves by approving of men, expressing their needs generously and enrolling men in meeting them, but many women are not yet able or willing to do that. They either fail to make the request, they make the request poorly, or they fail to reward their men with their approval and delight when the men have fulfilled their requests.

Our advice for women is to give up their anger at all the men who have failed them going back a hundred generations, give up the hope that men will ever behave like women, and instead accept men as the limited, but perfect creatures we are. Men were made for women, and women were made for men, we are each perfect for the other within God's plan. Women need to learn to approve of us and love us from where we are, and not from where they would like us to be. *"Lay down your sword"* says Alison Armstrong. I have only one disagreement with Alison, a friendly one: she thinks that women should lead this transformation, and I think that men could. But either one can make the shift, and the other will follow. Men create the shift by providing support, empathy and directness, by gaining emotional awareness and becoming more trustable. Women create the shift by clearing their anger and make-wrongs, by rewarding their men with their own happiness and forgiveness, and finally by amplifying that happiness through the request/appreciation cycle.

Men are designed as they are for a purpose, God's purpose is good.

When you and your feminine partners begin to get this, you will start to manifest the extraordinary power that masculine and feminine people can achieve by playing together on this field. You will start creating miracles in your life every day. Not just with your partner, but with everyone you meet. And you can start this process now, in this very moment, with every feminine person you meet. Take the lead as is your masculine duty, and also your joy. You do this by modeling servant-leadership and proactive loving, within your own masculine limitations. Some women won't get it, others will be annoyed, a few might even tell you to go fuck yourself, but you will likely score with most of them, and potentially big-time. They may resist until they get it – they *will* give you a hard time, and maybe even bust your balls, but when they get it, they will start to lead and from there the sky is the limit. When they begin to take back the lead, magic happens. And you can bask in their adoration, which you will have earned.

For all the reasons above, you need never apologize or be ashamed for being a man and for thinking and acting like a man. Just love as best you understand love, be true to yourself, and let the critics blow in the wind. You will be too busy loving to pay them any mind.

# PART 4: ADVANCED MAN/WOMAN

Advanced practices and distinctions start with the next Chapter: Feminism and the rise of **Whole and Complete**, which explains the current cultural context (some would say cultural disaster) of sexual relationships in the Western world. This part also covers the all-important topics of **Masculine Terms** (do this or die), understanding **Masculine Purpose**, the **Deep Feminine** and **Dark Feminine**, how to end a relationships, and more.

# 20 Feminism and the Rise of "Whole and Complete"

*"For men, love is a game; for women, it is all of life." – Tolstoy*

*"The emancipation of women thus degenerates into a mere counterpart to existing male structures." – Dieter Duhm*

One of the reasons that the idea of sexual polarity is difficult for many people to accept and embrace is that it challenges the dominant relationship model of Western-educated people for the last 40 years. This competing model could be called **Whole and Complete**. It developed from Women's Liberation, the human potentials movement, and all the way up to our contemporary gurus. In this chapter, I will do a brief analysis of why this happened. I hope to demonstrate to you that while **Whole and Complete** is an excellent idea when properly applied, many people, and especially men, will likely find it much easier and more rewarding to play **Man/Woman**.

## Whole and Complete: a brief history of women's emancipation

***Whole and Complete is the idea that to be fully in relationship you have to show up already healed.*** It is the idea that you cannot expect your partner to do things for you that you cannot do for yourself. You need to be primarily responsible for meeting your own needs. You can't ever fully depend on another person to meet your needs – and you certainly can never demand that. If you cannot meet your own needs for yourself, you have very little chance of being successful in relationship.

Before Whole and Complete came into vogue, our original relationship style of loving between a man and a woman was Sexual Polarity, or Man/Woman. It was never perfectly applied in any culture, instead it evolved naturally to more mature forms, up to and including the mediaeval concept of courtly love. Then the women's emancipation movements, starting in the late 1800's, killed it. The women were right to do so because sexual polarity had become institutionalized – it was serving as justification for attitudes, actions, and laws that were fundamentally disrespectful, depreciating, and disempowering to both sexes.

The institutionalization of sexual polarity was its death-knell, even though it took more than a century to die altogether. Incidentally this is the same error that many religions make: they try to institutionalize love. But love is too complex a phenomenon to become institutionalized. It's perilous even to attempt this. Remember Khalil Gibran: we must sometimes be *"wounded in our understanding of love."* Institutionalization passes rules and regulations in a futile attempt to make life wholly predictable, so that we may never be wounded. It doesn't work in the case of love, because sometimes we must do things for love that are entirely irrational and break all the rules. We can only be guided by our insides.

Women's emancipation, including women's lib, was necessary and timely. Even so, women's lib failed to deliver true happiness to either women or men. Sexual polarity went out of favor, except perhaps in American religious fundamentalism, which kept both the good and the bad aspects of the old model. Open the door for a woman or tell her she is beautiful? Sexist pig. Tell her you think you are better at solving certain types of problems than she is? How dare you! Not to mention your compelling desire to fuck everything that moves. You animal, shame on you.

Whole and Complete has many aspects, many of them positive, but here is one variant that can cause a lot of misunderstanding. The idea is that since we all must strive to become whole and complete, *men ought to be able to embody masculine and feminine traits equally, or at least learn how to mitigate the negative aspects of their masculinity.*

This is sometimes expressed as follows: **"Men: get off your obsession with fucking.** Sorry dude, but grow up, the times have changed. You need to transmute your sexual desire into something more holy and more respectful of her womanhood and of her feminine power. And if you wish to express it, you must do so in convoluted new-age language, or you are nothing but a caveman. You must love her deeply and tenderly except for the occasional moments when she too wants to fuck. Your failure to adapt will result in your being left behind by history. *The masculine gender has become obsolete, except for men who play by the new rules".*

Ouch. You might prefer to become a monk. Or maybe a soldier.

This idea doesn't seem to work for either gender. It is based on the delusion that men can change their essential nature. It's even possible that fucking her becomes your dominant thought the moment you lay eyes on her, taking over your brain and making you stupid. When that happens, your best and perhaps only move is to surrender. It's not a bad ride, really, after you surrender to it and to her. But whatever you do, do not make yourself small by pretending that you are something different than who you are. That never works in love.

## Man/Woman versus Whole and Complete

Let's compare and contrast the two relationship models. In general, **Man/Woman** is more in the nature of a negotiation ("reaching out" or "outer love," the masculine form of love), while **Whole and Complete** is more in the nature of unconditional love and acceptance ("reaching in" or "inner love," the feminine form of love). Of course this is a relative thing – you need to do both. But still, you should choose your primary game.

Whole and Complete is a wonderful model, but let me describe one of its more dubious aspects, as it relates to dealing with a feminine-polarity partner. The idea is similar to the one mentioned above, that men ought to embody feminine and masculine equally. Since this rarely happens, men are reduced to imperfect women who need to be fixed. It might be expressed like this: *You must be tender, loving and attentive to her, proactively sensing and responding to her needs, in one moment. And in the next moment you must let your passion take over and fuck her brains out. Depending, of course, on her desire or appetite of the moment, which you must intuit.*

Now, this is a lovely feminine sexual fantasy, harmless except when men are held up to it. And indeed it is harmful to women to be held up to men's sexual fantasies as well. This particular fantasy, however, has cost dearly both in terms of men's confidence and self-esteem, and in women's sexual satisfaction. The new standard judges men by a feminine standard. Since most men will not be able to meet this standard, applying it redefines men as **misbehaving women** [Alison Armstrong] who are continually disappointing and screwing things up – as in the caricatures of popular television.

This fantasy has been further affirmed (in its various ramifications) by the growth of pop psychology, New Age religion, and the "you can do/ be/have/become anything you want" movement. We are done with gender differences! Those things are for the older generation, while the enlightened young and chic pay no attention to gender difference any more. Just be yourself, and everything will be OK. Sexual relationships have become a flat playing field.

Oh. Really. I will believe "flat playing field" when I see men and women stop torturing each other. I am sorry, dudes of either gender, but look around you. How is this working out for you and your friends? Are you truly getting the love you want by "just being yourself"? Are you experiencing deep sexual intimacy? Are you living your life with the kind of purposefulness, deep satisfaction and joy that you know, at some level, you are capable of?

Whole and Complete is not wrong, **because in relationship everyone is right.** People have a good reason for being the way they are, and hence there is always something to agree with. *"Seek first to understand, and then to be understood"* [Stephen Covey]. I've found it helpful always to remember that in relationship everyone is right, in any kind of conflict with anyone, man or woman. That simple perspective – the granting to the other of human-ness equal to your own – could save both the relationship and your sanity.

Whole and Complete has aspects that are true and profound. Yes, we all need to heal ourselves. And there is a fundamental existential aloneness in the human condition that no partner can ever fully satisfy – only God can satisfy it, in the event you believe in a higher power or higher consciousness to the universe. Though men may be blinded by their obsessive fascination with women, the fact remains: **You are alone in the world.** It's you and God, if any. He is the only one who will go out with your last breath. Relationships are important for sure, but nobody will ever fully understand you and entirely meet your needs.

Even so, Whole and Complete looks to me to be a less powerful model, less useful and less effective toward the desired outcome of happiness and success, than the Man/Woman (Sexual Polarity) model. For most people, most of the time. This will not be true for everyone – some people are just not wired to play a sexual polarity game and will prefer to play Whole and Complete. Others will try to play a bit of both.

Victor Baranco describes it this way: you can play **Man/Woman** (Sexual Polarity) or **Man/God** (Whole and Complete). These are the two master games. Which one suits you better?

Man/God is another name for the best form of Whole and Complete and it truly is a fine game for those who can play it successfully. I will deeply admire you if you make the attempt. You can also play both games simultaneously. But most men will need to choose one as their primary. You just don't have enough attention to play two master games simultaneously.

### The problem with Whole and Complete (or Man/God)

Here is the big problem with betting all of your attention on the Man/God game: ***If you wait until you are fully healed or feel entirely "ready" to seek a partner or start playing with women, you may be waiting for a long time.*** Many people feel unable to commit to a relationship – or even to engage in an exploratory relationship, since our society does not provide any support for relationship models other than committed monogamy. Your fear of being hurt, in addition to the lack of socially acceptable alternatives, may make you afraid of engaging at all.

Only you know what is best for you, but you could be missing out on a lot of fun and transformation. *By choosing to hold back your love, you may fail to make a woman very happy – a woman who might be willing to accept you and appreciate you just as you are, with all your broken zones and rough edges.* She might find your broken zones kind of cute – or much less hateful than you find them. When you feel unable to commit to an evidently willing woman, think about this: Are you *sure* you want to preclude the possibility of being in authentic relationship with a woman because you don't "feel ready"?

Whole and Complete now rules the culture in terms of relationship models, even though it's probably not the best way for masculine people to go. Masculine people will usually want to develop themselves by reaching out and improving their awareness of other people and communication. Reaching out is inherently an expansive, or masculine process.

There is also the possibility that you imagine yourself as whole and complete but you really are not. You may be reasonably happy and productive in your life, a good citizen and well loved by many, but still feel that you are missing something. You may want a partner, but it's not happening no matter how many affirmations you repeat nor how much you troll Internet dating sites. You may wonder why you are still single and what's missing in you that prevents you from creating a relationship. These feelings may be especially real for feminine people. *"For men, love is a game. For women, it is all of life"* [Tolstoy]. This is less true than it used to be, now that women have careers, but it's still true. It is the very essence of male/female.

One possible reason that you are having so much trouble *may be that you may have not yet acquired the common sense to realize that you do have needs.* Needs that you cannot meet for yourself, only other people can meet them. You may be resisting the fact that you have a body. You are perhaps trying to meet these needs for yourself (or from God) but it's not fully working. God seems far away and he goes mute for days or perhaps decades at a time. Or perhaps it is working a little bit, but you are finding the road long and arduous. Twenty years of meditation and you still feel fucked-up in relationship.[9]

This can happen. If it's true for you, here is what I suggest: *get into the Man/Woman game.* Get into the game of loving women from where you are at, and not from where you would like to be. And then apply that same quality of love to yourself. *Loving yourself means accepting all your needs as legitimate, including sexual needs. All human needs are good.*

Whole and Complete generally breaks down on the bumpy road of sexuality. Unless you are a so-called **"spiritual athlete"** [Saniel Bonder[10]], it is possible that the attempt to process sexual energy through spirituality is going to be a losing game.

Your need for sexual expression is legitimate. It's also important for

---

9    See the work of Arjuna Ardagh (arjunaardagh.com/). After 20+ years as meditation teacher, he realized the greatest path of transformation is the path of relationship, and now coaches singles and couples on awakening in relationship.

10   See Saniel Bonder WAKING DOWN: BEYOND HYPERMASCULINE DHARMAS : A BREAKTHROUGH WAY OF SELF-REALIZATION IN THE SANCTUARY OF MUTUALITY. Bonder's breakthrough work is that there are two popular "Dharmas", Eastern dharma that teaches the unreality of the body, and Western Dharma that teaches the unreality of Spirit. Eastern teachers are "spiritual athletes" who succeed in renouncing their bodies and attempt to teach this to their students, who are typically unable to do this. Bonder teaches that human beings are both body and spirit, and that neither one can or should be renounced.

you to heed. My advice: accept that need and get on with playing Man/Woman.

One caveat here about playing Man/Woman, for men and women both: If you are repeatedly causing disasters in your relationships (rule of thumb: three times in a row within a year), then you do have to step back and reconsider. Just don't spend so long reconsidering that you revert to the other game, not yet whole and complete. As soon as you are done with your healing process, or at least starting to feel a little less crazy, get back in the game. Do it slowly if you want to, but before you feel completely ready. Be humble and be honest with you new partners in terms of who you are and where you are really at. You might create some magic for yourself and someone else, and surprise the both of you. You may already be more whole and complete than you realize. And your new woman might bring out the best of you, and your broken zones may no longer feel so overwhelming. They might just fade away on their own without your working so hard.

It might be good for you to take some attention away from yourself and give it to somebody else. And it may be very good for her to be the object of your love, however imperfect.

# 21 Masculine Terms

*"Women respond instinctively to strength. When a man stands up to a woman's nonsense, she knows he can protect her from her worst enemy: herself." – Alison Armstrong*

*I wanted to fight in order to be defeated... I was a power-woman and I longed to be tamed. I despised all these men who blushed in my presence because they were amazed or insecure. Men fell into great astonishment, then felt inferior, got complexes and hang-ups, and in the end I had to be their mother and build them up again and console them, which was contrary to my true nature." – Sina-Aline Geissler*

If you have made it this far, congratulations. What you have already learned is designed to give you some key concepts that could help you become not only the best lover that she ever had, but also her best friend. From here on, it is mostly practice.

There is, however, one missing piece. The knowledge you have acquired so far will be of limited value unless you become aware of your **Terms,** and you properly communicate them. If you don't do this you may bust your balls to please her and take care of her, you may give her more than any woman has a right to expect from a man, and yet she still won't be happy.

If she is not fully happy, the reason may be simple: *you are not happy with her.* If you are not happy, confident, powerful, and self-expressed, she will probably feel something is wrong. It may occur to her as her own failure, or something about her, that she cannot make you happy. Many women will blame themselves, consciously or not, if you are not happy with them. It may profoundly affect her self-esteem, and she may not even know why she is unhappy. For sure, you will hear plenty about all the things that are wrong with you, but this won't help either of you, because **she will not be telling you her deepest truth: that she yearns more than anything else for you to be happy with her.** And if you can't resolve this issue with her, you will probably eventually leave her, because few men can stick around forever with a permanently unhappy woman. We seem to be genetically programmed to work for them and try and please them, and we are similarly programmed to leave them when they cannot be pleased.

## Introduction to Masculine Terms"

So: *how* to do you decide and properly communicate your Masculine Terms? Getting it right goes to the heart of the game.

Let's go back to the prime directive: your commitment to supporting her. You might call this your Bodhisattva vow: *"May all women be happy, and especially my partner."* It is a total commitment, although within your value system. This concept refers to your time and attention, but also potentially to your money, resources, social network, and more. For best results, you have to be in all the way. Throw in all your chips. Double or nothing. Being in authentic relationship with a woman is going to take all you've got.

So, let's assume you understand that you are going to be a lot happier and more productive if you dedicate yourself to supporting her and following her lead. You have committed to her happiness and well-being. You are executing your Bodhisattva vow like a pro, and things are starting to go well for you, perhaps spectacularly well. You either have manifested a new partner and she is happy, or else your current partner has noticed your transformation. She may even be wondering how she could have ever missed the fact that you are a God. She may be feeling tender and raw, perhaps a little sad and emotional about all the years she wasted with you in conflicts and stupid arguments. She may still have good days and bad days with you, and may wonder whether this change in you is permanent, or whether you will soon go back to your old ways; but most likely she will be amazed and will be playing along with you – at least to the extent that she knows how.

But here lies the problem: *a woman – and particularly a woman in her power, such as you like – is going to continually test you until you say: STOP.* She may work you until you are exhausted and miserable and ready to kill both her and yourself. She may not be able to help herself from doing this, she would be violating her very nature. Indeed, ideally *she should not even try to restrict or contain the expression of her needs, no matter how insane to you – "you want whaaat???" It is actually not her job to restrict her needs and wants, or the communication of her needs and wants, based on how much she thinks you can handle. It's not her job to second-guess you or try and predict your capabilities, it's your job.* And if you fail to do this, both of you will be miserable: remember, she cannot be fully happy if you are not. It's in the nature of deep partnership, and especially for feminine people. *"If Mama ain't happy, ain't nobody happy."*

*If all goes according to plan, you will become her "project", in a way.* She will be serving you in this way. Indeed, you have to realize that in terms of raw emotional intelligence and processing power, you are like a child to her. You have an amazing intelligence, for sure, but it is unlikely that you will ever match her in the realm of your awareness of the emotional condition and relational intricacies of the people around you. You can try and meet her there, but it's a mistake to go crazy trying. You are better off just doing what you do brilliantly, and not interfering in what she does brilliantly.

This strategy is also known as **scaffolding** – you build the support structure around her building, and she does the same for you. I have heard it said: *"The masculine provides the banks, between which the feminine river flows."* This type of role specialization is the key to success. You are complementing and combining each other's different intelligences and processing styles to a common goal, in order to get a whole that is greater than the sum of the parts. The goal is your care for each other and for the world – that is, love, or greater inter-relatedness. *You are tapping in to one of the deepest and most powerfully transformational forces in the universe: sexual intimacy. The two of you together can create a happiness and power that neither of you alone has a chance to achieve.* This will, however, require some serious communication – and on both sides.

### So what exactly are your Terms?

Once you are clear on the game you are playing, you can begin to discern and express your own Terms. Here are some key distinctions that will help:

Yes, you want to support your woman to have all the love and success that she could ever want and more, and make her deliriously happy. *But you have needs that will not be met by her happiness alone.* True, many of a man's needs will be met simply by supporting her – producing or providing for her, and solving, or helping her solve, the life problems that she lays on you. This may include external problems like money, food, housing, and meaningful work, as well as internal problems to the relationship. As a masculine person, you actually love solving her problems, it's one of the keys to your happiness. You could consider yourself lucky that you have her problems to solve, or that you can solve together with her, as your life might be rather dull otherwise.

**But you can only take on so many of her problems in a day.** If you are like most men, you will also have a threshold in dealing with the **Dark Feminine**. And finally, you have your own purpose and mission in life that is not related to her, and which you cannot ignore.

So here is the thing: *she will continue to lay problems on you, give push back, show up as Dark Feminine, and generally give you a hard time until you say STOP.* She is not necessarily doing this deliberately. She is simply playing out her polarity, which you can enjoy and appreciate as much as possible – but only within your Terms.

Now remember – you do need to be thankful that she is laying problems on you. This is challenging you to greater consciousness, awareness, attention, and discernment. Solving her problems, or helping to solve these problems, makes your life richer, and responding lovingly to her objections is actually good for you too. It's not always easy nor quick to learn how to appreciate the Dark Feminine in her, but when you begin to see the brilliant results of your partnership you will get it. You will understand that this is how she operates and it is part of God's plan. **She is calling you to unconditional love.** She does this by continually testing you and your limits, and this is good. It's like free therapy. Forget about cult religions and spiritual leaders, let her be your teacher.

*But you also need to tell her when you have had enough.* Despite all her brilliant feminine discernment and ongoing attention on and awareness of you, she can neither fully know her desires except in relation to your feedback, nor fully know your needs until you tell her. There will come a time when you need to take the attention back on yourself.

*Telling her what you need, in masculine language, is called "setting your Terms."* It is an imperative necessity for you to succeed in relationship with a woman. It is actually the flip-side of her commands and requests. Her communication of needs and desires are slightly different since her needs are more fluid, changeable, and dependent on your response

– not to mention upended by her hormonal activity. Do be aware that "women's terms" are, in essence, her commands, which you will need to elicit, and which you will ignore at your peril. It's a two-way street.

### The problem of setting your Terms

There are two fundamental problems with setting your Terms, both challenging.

The first problem is that *you won't know right away how much you can take from her, what your limits are.* She will be laying problems on you and giving you push-back that challenges your self-concept and calls you to greater presence, awareness and attention. Be generous with her if you can: solve a few more problems than you are fully comfortable handling, and give her more attention than comes naturally to you. Strive to give her the benefit of the doubt, if you don't fully know yourself yet – as is inevitable. **You will discover yourself in relationship to her – that is her gift to you.** You will sometimes need to discern between your real terms and your superficial resistance to her. But when you get clarity on that, you need to speak up.

Which brings us to the second problem for men setting Terms: **You need to speak them and then back them up with action.**

Most men will have two types of Terms, soft terms and hard terms.

**Soft terms** can be expressed in a tentative way as an exploration of your relationship as soon as you become even dimly aware of them. You can say, *"Baby there is something I need to talk to you about. Something that I think I need from you (or that I am uncomfortable with in relation to you) but I am not fully clear yet and I need your help in figuring it out. Can you listen to me and then tell me what you think?"*

**Hard terms,** once stated, need to be backed up immediately with action: **You need to leave her if she fails to respect them, whether temporarily or permanently.** "Temporarily" could look like, *"Sweetheart I am really triggered by you right now and I just can't listen any more. I need space. I am very sorry that I cannot be here for you right now. I will be back."* This is a hard thing to do, because it may appear to you (and to her) that you are violating a basic commitment to your relationship and to being present for her. But in fact, honoring your own hard terms actually is serving her too, even when she does not see this immediately.

If it becomes very clear that she is not going to meet your hard terms, you may need to leave her permanently. See Chapter 27 for ideas on how to do this honestly and maybe even elegantly.

## Some examples of Terms

There are as many Terms as there are men. Here is a sampler.

A man's terms may relate to sexual or relational needs. You may want to make love to her, and in a certain way, and at some certain frequency. You may want to see her, or spend time with her, at a certain frequency: *"I need to connect with you and have a real talk at least every few days."*

Terms may relate to ways in which she is communicating with you, and attitudes she holds about you. You may need participation in joint expenses. She may have a certain attitude about you or a repeated communication pattern that just doesn't work for you. She may get depressed or be distant and unavailable to you, and it's approaching your threshold of what you are able to tolerate in a relationship. She may be miserable, angry, or uncommunicative more than you can receive. Her Dark Feminine may exceed what you can handle. She may treat you like an object, a money-object, sex object, or a taking-out-the-garbage object. You may feel unappreciated, disrespected or not listened to. She may have priorities that just don't work for you – her job, her friends and hobbies, her pets, her phone, her other lovers.

*If you don't communicate any of this, you are both screwed.* Remember: your masculine duty is to lead in communication. You must challenge her to have the hard conversations. It's possible she will avoid them, and you must also remember that you need to continuously elicit and support her greater self-expression, which is her equivalent of Terms. As you model for her how to responsibly set and enforce Terms or needs, she may reciprocate. You may even teach her a great lesson, since you may be better at this than she is, for both biological and cultural reasons. But if you fail to communicate your Terms and fail to elicit hers, you are both dead. Or almost: you will be stuck in an unhappy relationship, which is not much better than being dead.

It's possible that you feel your terms are completely unrealistic, or even unkind, and think that you could never ask her for that. *But you can – and should – ask her for anything that is important to you.* The worst that can happen is that you need to negotiate further, or even move on. Always ask for 100% of what you want and be prepared to negotiate the difference. And if you do need to move on, it's often better to do it sooner rather than later.

These are difficult concepts so I will risk a personal example. I had a partner who had some body-image problems. This is not uncommon for women – they can be extremely insecure about their bodies and obsessive about their weight. From the masculine point of view, this is ridiculous, since most men appreciate a woman with some curves. Most men appreciate the woman they are with, who accepts and approves of them, regardless of her body shape. So I had to make a Term: *"I am sorry baby, it doesn't work for me to be with a woman who hates her body. I love your body. I need you to get this handled. Go into therapy, find a 12-step program, go to a retreat, whatever. I am here to support you but you need to do this work."* You can say things like this to a woman! In fact, you *must* say to her what is true for you. You may not want to make a hard term of something like this example, but you do need to communicate *something*. It could actually be the best thing for her, a great gift to her. Without you, it's possible she could die still hating her beautiful body.

Note how this approach differs from asking someone to gain or lose weight. That's probably not going to work. Giving her a Term is one thing, it's quite another to lay a trip on her that she cannot win. But you can help her change her **mind-set** about her body.

Occasionally you may feel that you have communicated a Term to her but it's going nowhere. For example, she is chronically late or has no sense of the value of your time. It's possible that respecting this need of yours is impossible for her. By the way, the reverse may be true as well – she may have needs that are important to her, but impossible for you to meet without feeling bent into a pretzel. At some point you will need to decide if the term that you set really is a deal-breaker. There are alternatives to walking away: You can try and negotiate – again. You can try to set up protective systems. You can simply repeat to her what you want in the spirit of *"you don't need to get what you want if you can express what you want"* (See Chapter 40). You can give **Withholds** (see Chapter 37). Or you can stretch yourself and just let go of it. Enjoy playing with your phone while you are waiting for her, then enjoy her when she returns to your mutual project. Her priorities might actually lead to a better result than you expect. God works in mysterious ways. Express your ambivalence, maybe even your rage, but then let it go.

Alternatively, you can make a scene. A scene may make you feel momentarily better but don't expect permanent results and don't be surprised if it backfires on you. *"A man persuaded against his will is of the same opinion still"* [Benjamin Franklin]. It is quite difficult to change people even when they want to change, and if they don't want to, forget it. At best they will apologize and act contrite, and the next day they will be just the same. And the scene will likely be re-visited upon you in reverse until the accounts have come back into balance.

In Part 7 of this book, we give more communication techniques that can be helpful in resolving emotional tensions or needs conflicts.

# 22 What To Do When You Really Want to "Make Her Wrong"

*The essence of Eros lies in its power to violate and transgress social boundaries." – Dieter Duhm*

Setting your terms may incite all kinds of reactivity in her and maybe even activate her Dark Feminine. You may need to double your empathy, be discerning, and stretch. Being in relationship with a woman (or with anyone really) is rarely going to be easy or entirely painless. But you must stand your ground, for yourself and for the relationship.

Occasionally you will have really had enough and you want to leave her, temporarily or permanently. The natural human tendency is to **make her wrong** for this – have her be the reason that you are leaving her. In effect, you are looking for an excuse to leave her. ***Don't do this! You don't need to make her wrong in order to leave her!*** Instead, just leave because you want to, because the way she is being is not working for you, even as you freely acknowledge that there is nothing inherently wrong about how she is being. Sadly, it is human nature to make people wrong because we want to leave them, and of course it happens in reverse as well.

If you end up making her wrong for any reason, and you realize it, always apologize. Say: *"I am very sorry I made you wrong for ___"* or *"I made up a story about you because I was angry with you, that you acted condescending/disrespectful/selfish/arrogant towards me, and I want to apologize to you for that. It's not true and you did not deserve that."* And then reframe the matter as a *feeling or a need,* which is inherently not making her wrong. She cannot argue with a feeling or a need, provided that you truly present it as such.

It will be tempting to ladle a share of responsibility onto her for however you are feeling, but it will avail you little – suck it up, be gracious, and take the rap yourself. Admit your fault in the matter without demanding that she do the same: *"Baby I know I was an asshole with you,"* or *"Sorry, that was obnoxious."* Tell her how you felt, if you must: *"... but I felt really disrespected/ignored/unappreciated, I hate it when you get like this."* It may be better to just wait for her to ask you how you feel about the situation, or to apologize naturally. In general, take as much responsibility for your feelings and behavior as you can, promptly admit any wrong-doing or failures in communication, and apologize without excuses or delay.

*You want to do more than tell her how you want to be treated – you want to model it for her.* You do this by apologizing, promptly and wholeheartedly, even before she says anything about it, and without the demand that she do the same. Allow any insights about her own behavior that she may arrive at, to come in her own time. You are not her parent or her therapist. Of course if she never apologizes for anything, or is not prepared to listen to you, that may quickly become a hard term. But for now, just let her be. **To whatever extent she still triggers you, is the extent to which your work on yourself is unfinished.**

# 23 Dealing With Feminine Resistance: the Dark Feminine, and the Deep Feminine

*"Women are crazy, men are stupid. And the main reason women are crazy is that men are stupid." – George Carlin*

*"When it flows freely, love is the most profound and beautiful thing in the world. But when it is obstructed and betrayed, it is the darkest and ugliest thing in the world." – Dieter Duhm*

I have already discussed feminine resistance in Chapter 14. We also call this "push-back." This chapter goes even deeper, into the most extreme form of feminine resistance, which is the **Dark Feminine.** You want to greatly value any kind of resistance or push-back from a woman, for all the reasons already given, while at the same time *holding it lightly*. This is explained below.

To begin with, few women are trained to push back or assert themselves in the way that a man is. It is extremely uncomfortable for most of them and few are good at it, even some who think they are. If you are lucky enough to be with a woman who knows her own feelings and needs, and who can express negative emotion easily and gracefully, count your blessings. *And be sure to tell her how lucky you feel that she has such emotional clarity with you and is so expressive.*

You may feel initially dismissed or angry when she pushes back, but try looking at it this way: When she pushes back she is looking for internal clarification, and she needs your assistance for this. If you see that it's hard for her to talk about something, give her a big appreciation: *"I am so happy you are standing up for yourself around this issue."* And then listen carefully and reflect back anything you hear, understand or intuit. Stay with her until she is complete – *"thank you, is there more?"* – and then, if you have an issue or feedback, state it. However, stating your feedback will take the attention back onto you, so first repeat again what you heard her say and reassure her of your commitment, love and caring for her well-being and for her needs being met. Say: *"I have a deep desire to know all your feelings,"* or *"I am committed that you get what you need from this interaction."* Also mean it, and be prepared to demonstrate that. You demonstrate it by listening and by reflecting back what you are hearing.

Just saying the words is not going to be enough. If you are saying the words and she continues to respond negatively, that is a good clue that you are missing something. Double your empathy, or else say nothing at all. Or just let her words sit inside you, and let her know this: *"I am thinking about what you are saying to me, you may be right,"* or *"I am struggling to get you, but you may be right,"* or *"I don't know how to respond right now, but I am grateful that you trust me enough to say these things,"* or just *"I am listening, say more."*

Consider why she may be angry – it may not be about you at all. She may be having a bad day, or need a break from work, from the kids or from you. And then consider the clueless men she likely has had around her for most of her life – not to mention thousands of years of invalidation, oppression, rape and torture, some of which continues to this day. A great many men are simply clueless around women, not from bad intention but from ignorance. Indeed, ignorance is the usual (default) relationship between the sexes.

You may also get lucky. **It's possible that all she ever wanted was the thing that you are doing with her right now: appreciating, validating, and eliciting her feelings.** She may have never had this before with anyone, man or woman. She may calm down and become more appreciative of you.

*But even if she does start calming, she may not believe this is happening to her.* Never having experienced a man truly attentive and listening before, and operating from her internal doubt that a man could ever fully get her, she may doubt your sincerity. *She may think you are conning her,* and she may test you to make sure you are sincere. It's possible that she is right, you *are* conning her: maybe you just want to get her off your back so you can continue with your day. You may need to examine your own motives.

Your interaction with her could go either way. **It's also possible that nothing you can do or say is going to make a difference. She may just decide, or feel compelled, to go into her** Dark Feminine.

Now this is actually a great gift, but it may not immediately occur to you as such. For certain it is an offer that may well make you pause, since it's likely you will feel she is dragging you through hell and back – and for no reason that makes sense to you. But it is a great gift nonetheless.

## The Deep Feminine hunger

Many, many women want, more than anything else in the world, to love and be loved – and particularly, to be fully seen and received by a masculine person. That is the deep feminine hunger. But overlaid on this desire, for many, is a *despair* that such a thing is possible (it's the one thing she can't do for herself) and a fear, or maybe conviction that *she doesn't deserve it* – meaning she doesn't think she is good enough, attractive or smart enough. In other words, a woman will likely blame herself when she feels unloved – and she may feel that her life is ruined as a result. The one thing that she most deeply desires seems beyond her reach. It must be a truly dreadful experience to be female in a world of unconscious men who have no regard for women nor attention on them – men who appear to her to only want one thing, free sex, and who give out their love so stingily.

But don't feel too sorry for her, because all people (and women in particular, in their heart-of-hearts) sometimes like to *"go on an emotional ride"* and *"experience the full range of human emotions"* [Victor Baranco]. In a weird way, we humans sometimes enjoy negativity and even despair. I suppose it makes us feel alive and perhaps it's necessary to the full experience of our humanity and the discovery of our compassion. For some women, despair does seem necessary for the full emergence of her Deep Feminine, that brilliant beacon of love and light that men live and die for.

> **"BEING ON AN EMOTIONAL RIDE"**
>
> *This means to be experiencing strong emotion, alternatively positive and negative, and over a period of time. To call it a "ride" reflects a fundamental truth about people, which is that we like excitement, and that we create emotional situations both positive and negative for various internal goals, often unconscious, such as: wanting entertainment, challenge, growth, attention, drama, etc. Becoming more conscious of our internal motivations for wanting negative emotion is sometimes helpful.*

## Manifestations of the Dark Feminine

So what is **Dark Feminine** exactly? It's different for every woman. *But* *it is very likely that you will experience it as a targeted attack on all your vulnerable spots.* It's quite amazing how that works, and this is actually the value to you: she is calling you to greater self-awareness of your own garbage – in particular, to the arrogance and secret misogyny that most men in our culture carry. This is one of the reasons why the Dark Feminine is so challenging for men.

Some women go into Dark Feminine predictably, and severely, at a certain stage of their menstrual cycle – often three to five days before they start bleeding. If you are with such a woman, you may wish to put her cycle on your calendar, so you can be especially loving and attentive to her, kind and patient during this time – or else so that you can disappear for the duration. However, the timing and frequency of women's Dark Feminine is variable, and it can be triggered by anything. You will want to avoid major conversations and touchy subjects during the time your woman is in her Dark Feminine – whether it lasts a few hours or a week.

*Here is what it can look like:* great anxiety, anger and rage, depression, or sullen withdrawal. There may be tears, intense feelings of inadequacy, guilt or shame, self-hatred, or feelings of betrayal. She may be experiencing many different emotions all at once and voice beliefs and attitudes that seem utterly insane to you – even as you struggle to witness her experience without judgment. Her interest in listening to you and her openness to feedback may be reduced to zero. Indeed, your attempts to give her feedback may be perceived as attacks on her independent thinking, her judgment and her values. She will be throwing you curve-balls, and you will be catching them as best you can... which will likely not impress her.

**And to add insult to injury (at least from your perspective) it will all be your fault.** Pause here for a moment and consider that this might actually be true, *it is your fault.* It's possible, even likely, that the many insensitive and/or condescending things that you do or say to her every day, which she might ignore or forgive in her normal state, have suddenly become unbearable. It's also possible that she has just become absolutely clear that you are not the man for her and that it could never work between you – which of course is also your fault.

But regardless of the details, it may look to you that she has lost her mind. To the masculine mind, the Dark Feminine may occur as fear, or needing to be away from you for a time, or simply crazy. Tragically for everyone, *"crazy,"* or *"neurotic,"* or *"hysterical"* are the usual masculine dismissals of the Dark Feminine.

## So when facing the Dark Feminine, what do you do?

You say a prayer, ask God for strength, cover your balls and go on the **emotional ride** with her. Be with her in her negativity and despair – but without getting hooked in yourself. Be with her fully, but **hold it lightly** to the extent that you can.

If you sense that a woman wants to take an emotional down ride (*"sense,"* hah, the evidence will be compelling), you can accompany her there. Accompany her wherever she wants go, with your love and discernment. Follow her lead. Give her your full, undivided attention until she releases you – or until you purely can't stand it any more.

At minimum, when she seems to be riding ever downward, you can ask her directly: *"Are you wanting to go down with this right now?"* or *"What would it be like to go fully into your anger (or depression, or upset) right now,"* or even the most direct *"If you want to go into this right now, I can be with you."* This may occur to the masculine person as a strange thing to say, but most feminine people will instantly understand the question. The objective is to let her know you are with her. Over-communicate your love and appreciation for her as she goes through this process. Say to her: *"I have a deep desire to know all your feelings, including the negative ones."*

This is the meaning of *"holding it lightly."* It means to *"bear witness to:"* listen, appreciate, attempt to understand and empathize, but stay non-reactive. Don't take any of it too much to heart. Once she has calmed down – which she will, and the more attention you give her the faster it will go – then is the right time to discuss matters rationally.

If she is truly panicked and out of control, or utterly furious with you, you might start by reflecting that back: *"You sound really scared/angry/hurt."* You may imagine that she is overreacting or that the problem is insignificant but you cannot say this. Instead, avoid getting riled up yourself, and try to help her run off her **emotional charge**. Give her time to figure out what's really bothering her and what she needs. Remember the reason she is talking to you in the first place: She needs your help around her own emotional discernment and internal clarity.

It's not a man-bashing exercise for the sake of man-bashing – she probably would prefer to get back to loving you as quickly as possible. You can help her. Honor her right to think and feel as she does – it's in your best interest and if you can do this for her, it would be cruel not to. There really is a reason for everything she does, even if you cannot comprehend it with your single-focus brain.

This process may take quite a while and it may be difficult for you to hold back your brilliant analysis of the causes of her troubles and the simple solutions that you can see. If you absolutely must say it, do so, but be quick and get back to listening as soon as possible. However, usually it will be better to not say it, because you cannot fix it for her. If you are feeling *really* frustrated with her – to the point that you want to end the conversation – you might try saying something like, *"How can I win with you right now – what do you want from me?"* You might also say something like, *"Whoa baby, now I am totally confused. Slow it down for the dummy, what exactly do you want from me in this moment?"* Do not expect she will be able to give you an answer, she likely won't know or can't articulate what she wants from you in the moment; but it's possible she will be grateful for the question and the pause might help her. The more you can communicate that you are fine with her stormy process, and that you still love her, the quicker she will move through it. In the more likely event that you can't think of anything helpful to say, you might just look at her adoringly and with a tinge of concern and say something like, *"Thank you for trusting me enough to say these things."* That actually may be all she needs.

### Being entertained by the Dark Feminine

There is something else you should know in relating to the Dark Feminine. Something that may save your sanity.

***There is nothing wrong with being entertained by a woman's processing style.*** Of course, you won't tell her that you find her entertaining (because she might kill you), but you can allow yourself to be silently entertained by her. She is likely to rise much faster if you are non-reactive and she feels that you are fine with how she is being. Bringing yourself to where you can be entertained by her might actually keep you in a game that you would otherwise give up in despair – and thus it may serve you both.

Remember as well that whatever negative emotions that *you* feel, are going to be five times worse for her. Women judge themselves more harshly than men do. She may absolutely hate herself and how she is being. She may be in the dismal condition of not knowing whether she would be better off killing you or killing herself. Even if she is furious with you and you truly deserve it because you have done or said some dumb-ass thing, she may also feel guilty for being angry or upset and for taking up your attention with her problems. You may need to tell her directly, and repeatedly, that it's fine with you that she is upset and you are grateful that she feels safe enough to want to process difficult feelings with you. If you have even the smallest inkling that you deserve her anger, say so. Try saying: *"It's possible that I deserve your anger and if so I want to understand why. Please help me with this."* You probably d deserve it, but regardless it is best to assume you are guilty until proven otherwise in this type of interaction. Don't worry about it and trust that it will sort itself out.

*Welcome her anger, not just because you may deserve it, but because it may rock her world to receive your welcome and it may help her be complete quicker.* She may have never before been calmly received by a man. Your generous response may surprise and amaze her, and perhap shock her out of her anger in one second. Tell her you are absolutely committed to understand what you did wrong. You may even tell her how much you are getting out of her strength and beauty in this moment. You may want to tread cautiously here if she is truly furious with you – this is where the "Yes dear" or "I am listening" response may be best – but let her know non-verbally and make your being entertained by her look like love... which it truly is.

*Loving her and being entertained by her have the same root: your delight in her and in her company.* Just don't lose compassion in your entertainment – you must hold both simultaneously. Talk to her of you attraction and devotion to her – she needs to hear it now more than any other time. Tell her what she wants to hear: that she is important to you and that you care for her, no matter how she behaves. Even if it's not fully true in that moment, say it anyway, at least to the limits of your value system. Saying it will help make it true, because *"Love is an intention"* [Jerry Jud]. Say it between clenched teeth if you must, but sa it. Say: *"I have a deep desire to know all of your feelings, and I love that you trust me enough to say all these things."* Keep that perspective, even those exact words, on a card in your wallet, in case you forget them.

## Keys to the Kingdom

*Remaining engaged in the face of the Dark Feminine is the key to the kingdom in relating to feminine people.* Everybody loves a happy woman. Loving an unhappy and/or angry woman is more challenging, but the results are simply going to blow you away. She may be eating out of your hand within the hour if you do this right. She may also feel quite sexual afterwards – many women do after they have unloaded negative feelings, when they feel heard and received. Stretch. Do your masculine duty, which is to provide witness consciousness and non-reactivity. *This is the hero's journey and you are already 90% there. Don't give up now. It's actually easier for you (due to your brain structure)* to be non-reactive than it is for her. Give her that, to fail to do so when you are able to, would be both cruel and stupid. Help her get out of "fighting" and into "fucking" – by making love to her verbally through your acceptance of her and your surrender to her process. This is what both of you wants.

Of course, whatever you do must remain within your value system. If you have truly had enough you need to say so and, at the limit, take a break. Ideally you will promise to come back soon. You may feel really hurt and angry, and you may need to take space for a while – same as she does. You may feel so battered and bruised that you can't even talk about it, not right now. This is fine, just let her know that you need a break and that you *will* be coming back.

# 24 Delving deeper into Masculine Purpose

*"A woman does not want to be number one." – David Deida*

The idea of **Masculine Purpose** is fundamental to masculine sexual polarity, but it can also be very confusing. The most compelling expression of this idea is from David Deida. I recommend that you read some of his books (see the Bibliography Chapter). I also believe, however, that to approach Deida's ideas with an uncritical eye is dangerous – as he would agree, no doubt. Here are some of the limitations of Deida's thinking where practical man/woman relationships are concerned.

## David Deida: a critical review

Deida speaks very eloquently on the practice of sexual polarity and Tantric sex as a path to enlightenment. His books have been profoundly inspirational to me. I view them as the first modern and compelling articulation of the relationship style called **Sexual Polarity**. Practicing sexual polarity essentially involves responding to your partner in a way that meets her deep needs for growth, connection, pleasure, and awakening – needs that will be different from yours as a masculine purpose. It is a very high form of loving.

Deida believes that for a man's life to be a true expression of his deep love for women and for the world, he has to be aware of his purpose, or mission, and he needs to be living from that awareness or consciousness at all times. This is a profound truth, but also controversial because it requires that a man's purpose be more important than any single relationship in his life. It means, essentially, that to a person living in masculine polarity, his woman is replaceable. If his woman is no longer fundamentally serving his purpose, he must leave her, or else risk losing both his purpose and his woman – since eventually she will leave him anyway, or else she will make his life hell until he ends up leaving her. I believe Deida's analysis to be correct.

The problem, however, is this: ***Loving a woman tends to be a full-time job.*** Certainly a man needs his purpose, this is central to the full expression of masculine consciousness, and without it he is lost. But a woman who is deeply engaging her polarity and in her feminine power – the power to fully embody the flow of love through her, and the power to endlessly fascinate and motivate men – such a woman is unlikely to be fully gratified by a man unless she feels that he has his full attention on her when she needs him. To be fully successful in a sexually polarized relationship, a man will need to pay attention to his woman when she wants him, and not only when he is not otherwise occupied with his purpose, or feels like giving her some attention. The needs and demands of your woman may well seem to take you off your purpose, at least for a while, and sometimes, you will need to surrender to that. In fact, unless you can get physical separation or live apart, you may have no choice but to surrender. Your surrender may need to be total, although always within your value system. It is possible here that *"half-measures will avail you nothing"*.

If you are unable or unwilling to fully surrender to giving your woman love and attention when she needs it, it's possible that things will go better for you with multiple sexual partners, none of whom is primary. This may not be practical for many people, however, because it does not fit conventional relationship structures such as monogamy. It's also possible that your partner, or partners, are fully satisfied with you sexually, maybe even to the extent of being addicted to you sexually, but unfulfilled in other aspects of their relationship with you. This is likely not a winning game, and you may be continuously changing sexual partners and/or dealing with feminine drama and Dark Feminine, or investing a lot of energy in developing new relationships that don't last long. This will likely take you off your purpose and ultimately be self-defeating.

A man will be happiest with a woman who is fundamentally aligned with his purpose, one who is able to accept him as he is including all the limitations of his attention. But sometimes he will have to surrender to her need for love and attention even when doing so takes him away from his purpose. A woman needs a lot more than sexual love and attention from a man. She wants you contributing to her in all the ways that you are capable of. That is what love is.

The tension between a man's purpose and his woman's desires can be a difficult problem for which there is no easy answer. If you follow the main ideas of this book, which is to approach everything as a negotiation, and provided you are able to exercise deep listening and empathy, you will be much more likely to succeed. Sometimes, however, there is just no winning. Either you surrender to her and feel unfulfilled and resentful, or you set limits with her that don't work for her and you pay for it later. Deida seems to suggest that a man should always choose his purpose over his woman. It's not that simple because for many men, love of women is core to their being and to the value that they can offer to the world. It feeds them deeply and therefore is central to their purpose. You must be able to discern whether a woman deeply needs you in the moment, and you giving her that would transform you both – even when you are having a crisis at work, or you desperately want to write your blog – or whether she is simply testing you. This is difficult.

Deida says that a woman does not really want to be number one. This is true and also not true. She does not want you to give her anything that you do not truly want to give – she does not want you to betray yourself. You need to have Terms and they need to be communicated and enforced. But sometimes you will need to stretch. Your woman will cause you to stretch – that is her job. Unless your relationship with her is primarily sexual, and you are not necessarily meeting each other's everyday intimacy and connection needs, you must honor and carefully consider her request for you to stretch your boundaries, even to the point, sometimes, of dropping or adapting your Terms. Your surrender to her must be as complete as you can manage. The more surrender you can manage, always within your value system, the more transformative will be your relationship.

I sometimes feel that for Deida, a man's purpose is like God: to be unconditionally obeyed. That is only likely to work for a man who has made a total commitment to a spiritual life or to a career goal and is willing, if necessary, to live without women. Most men are not willing to do that – not unless there is truly no other way. There usually is another way. A way of deeper love and of deeper negotiation. Women call us to that, and we should heed their call.

If you resonate with this, if you feel that you *"love and must needs have desires"* [Khalil Gibran], then you may need to practice deep discernment in this area, as well as deep negotiation.

Note that Deida is not wrong. The difference between his ideas and mine is one of emphasis. Deida's primary interest is in the physical and spiritual dimensions of love between a man and a woman, and particularly in the transformational possibilities of the sexual act itself. My emphasis is on the emotional or relational aspects of love between a man and a woman, which can certainly include deeply transformative sex. My point is that for most women, you have to get the emotional and relational issues handled *before* you can have deep sex. You have to do your negotiating. Skipping directly to Sacred Sexuality will only work if your woman is in agreement, if that is what she wants and is ready to receive.

We return to this topic in Chapter 33: Sacred Sexuality.

# 25 Educating Yourself, Teaching Her to Ask for What She Wants, and Avoiding Pitfalls

*"If we were to wait for our desires to be fulfilled before we began living, we would probably never begin living." – Dieter Duhm*

## What if your woman is not asking you for anything?

Here is another common problem, and particularly with younger women: *Your woman is not asking you for anything.* If she is not asking for anything, and yet appears happy, you may wonder, what is the problem? It may sound strange to you that her being *"too nice"* or *"too compliant"* could be trouble. And yet it can be.

This situation is similar to women's tendency to over-please – an aspect of having poor boundaries (see Chapter 29). It may be quite fun for you for a while, but you are heading for a certain let-down or betrayal, because *you cannot possibly understand and anticipate all of her needs.* Remember also that *her natural feminine condition is to lay problems on you until you tell her to stop.* If she is *not* laying problems on you, it's likely she is not occupying her feminine polarity, and the relationship will fail. You would need to play another game with her – or else you will both be paying for this, in tears and betrayal, a short distance down the road. It may also be that she is lying. Women do choose to lie sometimes. It can be terrifying for her to share her true feelings when she believes these might hurt you, upset you, or cause you to leave her.

The situation in which she is not expressing her needs should be resolved as soon as possible, for everyone's sake. It's possible that you are not inviting her self-expression and commands sufficiently strongly. Or else, she may just be inexperienced in relating to men (or perhaps she is lying). *You need to cut this off at the gate, or it will come back to haunt you.*

***She is not serving you or her by being too nice.*** When she is being too nice she is essentially in an unspoken (and unholy) contract with you: that you will like her so much that you will want to intuit what she wants and then give it to her. That does not work with men! She needs to mature into her true feminine power, which is expressing her needs and enrolling you in meeting them. She needs to find her real boundaries, firm up her value system, and learn to self-express or assert. Failure to do this is inviting disaster. *If she fails to speak up, it will be your fault – I am sorry but this is just the reality.*

It is virtually impossible that a woman will be happy for long if she doesn't express her needs. If she is head-over-heels in love with you and you can do no wrong, that is good, and you will want to extend this fortunate but temporary condition as long as possible. You do this by encouraging her self-expression and trying to move her toward a more mature relationship with you. And also congratulations – you must be doing something right that she is so in love with you. Of course this could be caused by your good looks, easy wit or debonair ways – this is still good, but don't get complacent, or you will likely have a steep fall. Be proactive. Re-double your efforts and ask her a lot of questions.

## The many pitfalls of relationship

To be successful in relationship, women need to approve of their partners, express their needs generously, and enroll their partners in meeting them. But few women know how. And few men are capable of maintaining the ongoing attention and appreciation of their partners to the degree that is necessary to fully gratify most women. The risk of failure in relationship is high. And so you would be wise to start thinking of yours and your woman's education as soon as you start to get serious with each other. Since relationships are so difficult, you will want to start working on your partnership at the earliest opportunity. It may be much harder later.

How do you do this?

*First of all, through the prime directive: Commit to supporting her.* Let her know you value and are awaiting her spoken desire, and then demonstrate your responsiveness to that. Once she is engaged, make sure that she knows that she has your attention and that you will do pretty well anything she wants, provided it be within your value system. Ask her directly what she wants. If she is not sure, or can't come up with ideas, give her a menu: *"We could do X, Y or Z right now. Which do you prefer?"* She will appreciate you for that.

You may need to set a **hard term** here. Tell her that her self-expression is a condition of your relationship, and to stop being a little girl and start behaving like a woman. Tell her directly that you expect her to tell you what she needs day and night. Give it to her straight – you may as well bust her fantasy now that you are going to respond to unspoken needs. Tell her to ask you nicely for what she wants if she can, and if she can't, to ask you anyway.

You can also teach her to give **Withholds** (see Chapter 37) or ask her to practice **Non-Violent Communication (NVC)** with you. NVC is more than conflict resolution, it's about identifying and articulating needs.

Beyond these suggestions, you are going to need help. You cannot help a woman mature into her full power and self-expression all by yourself. You need help, particularly from her sisters, and perhaps from people who do this professionally. Make sure you support her relationships with her girlfriends, and encourage her to attend workshops on relationships and sexuality (see Chapter 41: Training organizations). Go with her to these workshops, whenever possible – they could be a wonderful experience to share with her, and will likely open up your communication tremendously. Take her to a Shalom Mountain couple's retreat, it will likely blow both your mind and hers. Do a workshop with Alison Armstrong, attend the Landmark Forum together, find an NVC class or retreat. Do whatever calls you, but do something. ***Don't just wait for problems to come up and then ask the Good Lord to save you both from your ignorance and laziness.*** Be proactive, love must be cultivated like the most beautiful and fragile garden. It requires continuous attention. ***Do your masculine duty of leading in action and communication.***

If all this occurs as a lot of work, remember this: playing the Man/Woman game successfully, and with full heart, will utterly transform you both. Most of the good things in life do require a little work.

# 26 Handling Disinterest or Lack of Attraction

*"Men and women are sexually attractive because they possess an erotic self-awareness." – Dieter Duhm*

A woman may be lacking attraction, commitment, or is communicating indifference to you – while maybe still letting you see her or even fuck her. Or perhaps she just wants a fuck buddy and you want more. This is unlikely to be a healthy situation for either of you. You *may* be able to do something about this. This chapter explores some options.

It used to be that the majority of commitment-phobes were men, but that is no longer the case. Women may lack commitment as much as men, but sometimes they will pretend otherwise. They may pretend they really want a relationship, but then lay down a list of requirements that Superman does not meet (*he lives with his mother, right? Cut*). *To be successful in relationship you have to do the work.* It can be the most rewarding work you will ever do, but sometimes men and women both are reluctant to take it on because they are afraid they will fail and will be hurt. This generally indicates a lack of self-confidence in relationship to the opposite sex, often a result of painful experience. Many people have simply given up on relationship and sexual intimacy. *"Once hurt, twice shy."*

The problem may be compounded by social conditioning and misinformation, and/or broken cultural norms that don't work. Men and women both may attempt to take on relationships Hollywood-style, and fail. Very few people know or understand the kind of deep personal work that is necessary to enter into true partnership and achieve deeply fulfilling sexual intimacy. Nor the extraordinary happiness and power that is possible to achieve by doing this work. They have, perhaps, been *"wounded in their understanding of love"* [Khalil Gibran] and as a result, they have quit.

It can be difficult and painful to attempt to engage a person of either sex who appears indifferent to you or is unwilling to commit, especially when you are strongly attracted to them and see tremendous potential in the relationship. But you should not take it personally. Sexual intimacy is the deepest and hottest crucible of personal transformation available to you or anyone. Not everyone is ready for it. You may not be ready for it either. You will know this because you continue to attract emotionally unavailable partners. In this case, as indicated in Chapter 20, you may want to return to playing Whole and Complete for a while – that is, heal yourself.

***Approach all relationships out of a sense of your own value and contribution.*** Your making yourself transparent to other people – revealing your need without shame and being vulnerable – is a great gift to them, as it gives them the opportunity to do the same. If you are not certain that your revealing your need is actually a gift to them, if you don't feel this in your bones, perhaps you need to heal this in yourself. See the Training Organizations and Bibliography chapters for ideas on how to proceed.

### How to respond to indifference or lack of commitment

So let's assume you are aware of your own value, are prepared to let her know what you want, and you are ready to do the work. Here is how you might respond to indifference or lack of commitment from a woman.

*The first reason why a woman may be indifferent to you is that you are simply not the man for her.* It's possible that you find her stunningly attractive and clearly visualize your brilliant life and deep happiness together, but she does not see it your way. You are doing your best with her but you are just not getting acceptance. You feel like you are pushing a boulder uphill. Here is what you do: *Just let her go.*

If you think she is playing a game with you, consciously or not, you can easily test her indifference by telling her that the relationship is not working for you, and why: obviously she doesn't care for you, so why should you hang around? (Subtext: There are so many other beautiful women hungry for your love and for that sweet-talking tongue of yours. Not to mention your deep understanding of feminine psychology and exquisite sexual technique). If she objects, you have something to talk about – this is a perfect time to set a Term, or better yet, share a kiss.

*A second possible cause of her lack of commitment could simply be that she is in resistance.* In which case you could just put more attention on her, and lay on the compliments and appreciations. Work with her as you would with any woman: love her as best you can. You would, however, need to use your discernment (intuition) to know which is the true cause: that she truly doesn't care for you, or that she is fighting her attraction or own self-worth issues. Maybe you just need to give it more time for more shared fun and experiences. Or maybe she just hasn't yet considered the benefits of being with you, or doesn't yet trust your motives and character. It could be any number of things.

You may get an opportunity to ask her directly why she is indifferent to you. Ask her what you do or how you are being that puts her off. The answer is certain to be valuable to you, whether you choose to act upon it or not, and whether you end up together with her or not.

## What to do if she tells you she is not attracted to you

If she tells you she is not sexually attracted to you, don't take it too much to heart. Sexual attraction can often be created even when not initially present, especially in women, so this could be what's called a **Story**. She may have a "story" that she is not attracted to men of a certain type, for instance, or that she herself is unattractive, or that she is doomed to fail in relationship, etc. It's also possible that she is just trying to slow you down and that she wants you to get to know her in a non-sexual (or non-dating) way. If you are brave, you can ask her how unattractive you actually are to her, and why. It's not impossible that you can do something about this, either immediately or over time, as in becoming more fit – she may give you a push in a direction that you want to go anyway. You could ask her if there is any chance at all – even a tiny chance – that she would ever make love to you. Unless the answer is a categorical *"No, never,"* you may want to continue to play with her. You don't have to take as gospel her telling you she is not attracted to you.

> ### *"STORIES"*
>
> *A "Story" is a belief or judgment we make about a situation which may be wrong, limiting or disempowering. People create beliefs, or "Stories" from their experiences, which may be true or false or both. To call these beliefs "Stories" highlights the fact that beliefs are really just an overlay on a complex reality, and that changing our stories is often the only thing needed to begin to experience our lives in a radically different way.*

The same rule applies to the famous *"let's just be friends"* response. Listen to her and agree with her, but don't necessarily give up on her. Few feminine people are entirely indifferent to the laying on of compliments and appreciations when they are coming from an authentic place. If you think she is a Goddess, and you let her know this subtly or overtly, and just hang out with her while responding to her and making pleasurable offers for fun, food, or whatever, there is no telling what could happen. If you are bold, and think she might be receptive, you may try offering her a **Sexual Research Date** (see Chapter 30) with a clear agreement of no strings attached. You may also just continue to put out love energy in all directions, attract other women into your life, and when she sees you with other women who are responding to you, realize that she loves you and wants you after all. All this may take time, so don't quit too soon especially if you feel a real connection.

# 27 How to End a Relationship

*"The goal of relationship is not longevity."* – Victor Baranco

Sometimes, you will come to the end of the road with a woman. You may run out of time or patience, just feel that you can't handle her any more, or she is telling you by her words and actions that she is done with you, or does not love or care for you any more. Or maybe you have tried everything, have doubled your attention and your empathy but it's just not working. Maybe she is not meeting your hard terms. You have communicated clearly, listened deeply, and it's still not working. You *"just can't get no satisfaction"* [Mick Jagger]. It's time to give it up.

You need to leave her. It's sad, but necessary. It is the loving thing to do – let her find another guy who can handle her better than you. Leave her as nicely as you can and without making her wrong. Don't knock yourself, either. It happens to everyone.

Breaking up is tough, especially after you have invested significant amounts of time with her, and even more so after you have children and businesses and property together. It can be an extremely painful and drawn-out process. Do the needful: Seek closure, lick your wounds, do some personal healing, apologize for what you did wrong in the relationship (increase your empathy), but then get on with your life. It is the right thing to do – indeed the only thing to do. *Imshallah* – it is God's will. Remember: nobody fully understands the reason that relationships form and dissolve and their karmic purpose. Love is ineffable, and will from time to time *"shatter your dreams as the north wind lays waste the garden"* [Khalil Gibran]. You are not always in control. But if you have any belief in God or a Higher Power, you can trust that these things happen for a reason and for the greater good of all. Play your part and be humble. Then get up off the floor and love again.

You would be wise to over-communicate with her during the time before and after you leave her – make it about you, not her. You do this by not making her wrong (see Chapter 22), while assuring her of your love, affection, respect and gratitude – to the extent that this is still true for you, of course.

It is possible you will be in a big hurry to leave her, you have just had enough. You may simply be drained or have nothing more to give. It has stopped being fun with her, and other projects (and maybe other women) are calling you. You may need to slow down the process, both for her sake and yours, as much as possible and always within your value system. However, try not to lose yourself in the process and don't let it take forever. When you are done, you are done.

In slowing down the process, remember that the quality of your next relationship can be set by how well you loved the one before and how well you reached closure with her. If at all possible, assure her that you will always be her friend and are available to her for whatever she needs, within the limits of your value system. Continue to be her friend, and love her, as best you can, even though you cannot be in relationship with her, or she with you.

If you have become repelled by her, you would need to ask yourself: *"What did you like about her in the first place?"* And then return to that anytime you relate to her. Even if you have made a disaster out of it, you may be able to return to where you started with her (that worked, presumably) any time you want. If she will allow it.

***A relationship with a woman is never really over.*** You will carry her (and her teaching) with you for the rest of your life, and if you are wise, you will be grateful that, for a time, she graced you with her love and you were her man. Maybe a night and maybe a lifetime, but she blessed you during that time. *The love of a woman lasts forever. It is never truly wasted or lost.*

# PART 5: SEXUALITY

In this section we cover attitudes and practices most likely to satisfy a woman sexually. We begin this part by looking at the cultural reasons for women's low degree of sexual satisfaction the world over, and what can be done about it.

# 28 Human Sexuality 101: the Sea of Misinformation

*"We have (falsely) learned that sexuality is a matter of the heart and not something that can be the object of intellectual exploration." –*
*Dieter Duhm*

Sexuality is one of the greatest gaps between men and women and where some of the greatest differences emerge. It is also an area of great ignorance and misinformation for many people.

Due to the enormous diversity of sexual needs and appetites, it is challenging to provide sexual advice that doesn't come across as trite, or even wrong. Generalizations of what men and women want in relationships are already suspect, but generalizations of what we want in sex are nearly impossible. For example: I can say that women want attention and sincere appreciation, and be right 90% of the time. But it is impossible to say how 90% of women want to be made love to, as there is no such thing. All I can do is provide some general guidelines, or pointers on sexual techniques and sexual communication practices that are likely to be useful. But you must use your own discernment, add to this information that you already know about yourself and your woman's sexuality, and finally, take everything with a critical eye. Be guided by your intuition and by your woman's felt needs and communications. Indeed, **the most important success factor in your love-making is not technique. It is your presence,** or attention on and responsiveness to your sexual partner.

Notwithstanding this, I am still going to offer you a "sexual program" that is likely to help you succeed with most women, at least as a starting place.

The basic technique I will attempt to teach you – to the extent that these things can be taught in a book – is called a **Do-Date.** This is a type of manual stimulation of the clitoris, sometimes called a "yoni massage." The Do-Date technique is based on Victor Baranco's four decades of research on female orgasm and man/woman relationships. It is a proven technique that leads to most women having orgasms, and often very satisfying ones. Female orgasm, needless to say, is a wonderful thing that has all kinds of health and psychological benefits to women. is also, in many cases, essential to the health of your relationship.

Having your partner achieve satisfying orgasms with you is not the only goal. Women have all kinds of needs, most important of which, for many if not all women, is to feel seen, appreciated and cherished by yo. Women want to feel your emotional presence and your caring for then Sexuality is just one area of your caring for them, albeit a very importa one. Mastering the art of female orgasm will put you ahead of the game for sure, and can be very fun for both of you, but it is only the beginnin of the Man/Woman game, and of your work with her.

Clitoral orgasm through manual or oral stimulation is, for many wome a very satisfying type of sexuality. It is also an excellent way to begin a sexual relationship, maybe even the best way to begin, provided she agrees of course. *However it is only one way to go about things.* You can talk to her about this, ask her what she wants, what she likes. Begin a sexual negotiation with her.

If you follow the instructions below, you will be ahead of at least 50% men. And maybe 90%.

**The sexual facts aren't pretty**

Statistics show that only about 65% of women (two out of three) experience regular orgasms with their partners. But due to the complexity of women's sexuality, the fact that women's sexuality is not men's forte, and the fact that women are often not self-expressed around their sexual needs, we can probably assert that *no more than half of women are fully sexually satisfied with their partners.* It is also a fact that only about 25% of women experience orgasm through intercourse alone.

What makes the situation worse is that many women may say they are sexually satisfied, when they are not. This may be because they are no able to face the truth, but more likely it is because they have nothing t compare it to. A woman who is enjoying regular orgasms with a man she loves and who she feels loves her, may be utterly transformed by t experience. Sometimes you can tell just by looking at her whether she coming regularly. There will be a bounce in her step and a radiant aur about her. She may come across to you and everyone else as this big bubble of love, joy and delight, which is her natural Deep Feminine sta

*And yet, despite the reality of men's poor sexual performance, most men imagine that they are great lovers.* Do this experiment: directly ask your male friends whether they think they are good lovers. Do you think that half of them will confess to fearing they are not very good in bed? And yet, this would be women's honest assessment – women being, of course, the arbiters on this question. *"Not very good in bed"* should not be taken as a put-down – women are complicated and their sexuality even more so, it is a miracle that good sex happens at all – but it is still a sobering thought that half of men lack either the knowledge or the skill to fully satisfy a woman. For sure, men are becoming more aware of women's sexuality and better at serving their needs, but there is still a big gap. Even men who do have good sexual technique may have little presence, and/or may be missing fundamental information about feminine psychology in sexual situations (see the next chapter on **women's over-pleasing**).

Some men also doubt their ability to sustain an erection long enough to please a woman, or they may harbor fears about the size of their penis. Fortunately, this is not an issue.

Sexuality is a vast and infinitely interesting subject. You can learn more by taking courses and doing your own further research – see the Training Organizations for a list of sexual educators, and the Bibliography. There is truly no end to this study, should you apply yourself, particularly if you become interested in Sacred Sexuality (see Chapter 33). Sacred Sexuality, sometimes known as Tantra, is a different approach than the one presented here. I strongly suggest you explore it, but I also suggest you begin by learning the basic clitoral orgasm technique. Once you have mastered the basic **Do-Date**, and your woman is coming well, you can move on from there as per her direction and/or your mutual interest. You can have an infinite amount of fun with this.

### So – why are women sexually unsatisfied?

There are three fundamental reasons why women are sexually unsatisfied.

- First, women and men alike are untrained and uneducated about the sexual practices that would really excite them and lead to fulfillment.

- Second, women lie, or fail to tell their whole truth. It can be hard enough under normal circumstances to elicit a woman's deep needs.

It is doubly hard in matters of sexuality – matters that lie so close to the deep feminine heart. She just won't tell you, and often she can't tell you. Women are afraid that they will hurt our feelings, or even that we will leave them if they tell us the truth. In fact, the more she likes you and wants you, the harder it may be for her to tell you the truth about what she wants in bed, and what you are doing, or not doing, to satisfy those needs.

- Third, men may take very poorly to sexual direction, and/or are uneducated in sexual negotiation. We are, many of us, overly identified with our sexual performance, we see it as an aspect of our manliness, and therefore take poorly any negative feedback from women.

The lack of women's self-expression in matters of sexuality is a huge challenge for men. It is not a problem that can ever be fully solved, as men and women can only fully know themselves in relation to the other, and so we cannot expect women to fully know their desire without our help. The problem is that men are not always of great help. It is the blind leading the blind.

Notwithstanding this, basic knowledge and techniques covered in the next few chapters could make a big difference.

# 29 Women's "Over-Pleasing"

*"While women can find almost anything, we are challenged in finding our True Selves. And, after we've found it, it's easily misplaced in our compulsion to please, produce and take care of others." – Alison Armstrong*

Once they have accepted you, most women will want to please you sexually. They may want this badly – they will want you to be happy with them, for reasons both genetic and cultural: Women are trained from birth to derive their value from their ability to attract and keep a man.

*The problem, is that out of a desire to please you, she may become willing to do almost anything to keep your love, including acts that lie outside her value system and are just wrong for her.* She may also lie about her orgasm, or fake orgasms. She may have given up on her own sexual pleasure, and just want you to be done as quickly as possible. *You do not want this.* You do *not* want a woman to do anything sexually that she doesn't want – and you obviously don't want her to lie to you. You want her to enjoy and appreciate her sexuality as much as you do. *You want sexuality to be a joy for her, not a chore, an obligation, or a source of conflict or tension to her.*

Doing sexual things with her that she doesn't really want is not a loving thing to do. If she is not comfortable and secure enough to be truthful with you, she may accept, or even offer to do things that she doesn't really want to, but this will make her unhappy. She will not say anything, or even necessarily be aware of it

> ### *"COMING FROM HER SURPLUS"*
>
> *This is when a woman offers sexual play that you want (but may not necessarily be what she desires for herself) from a sincere place of generosity and desire to give to you, rather than a sense of guilt or obligation towards you, or fear that you won't like her if she doesn't do it. For a woman to do this, she usually has to be fully sexually fulfilled herself first – she needs to be "coming from her surplus," not from scarcity.*

until afterwards. However, she will be angry, at both herself and you, and you will pay. She may become sexually withdrawn, make you work much harder to get her into bed next time, or act irritable and bitchy.

I know this is unfair. You may think she did whatever it was of her own accord, or maybe in response to an honest request from you. And you would be right, but so what? Being "right" with a woman will never serve you. For both hers and your own good, you need to preempt this situation at the outset or it will come back to haunt you both. It is also possible that she may have honestly wanted to please you, but is now overcome with sexual shame. You really can't know what is going on inside her head, and you can't depend on her telling you. For this reason you need to be hyper-vigilant to the problem of **women over-pleasing**, and to the issue of women's sexual boundaries.

The more she does for you out of a desire to please you, or from a fear of losing you, the more angry she is going to become. And she probably won't quite know why. And this is tragic, because her anger is likely to drive you away – when she actually wants the opposite, more attention from you. The flip-side of women wanting men to act like women, is men expecting women to act like men – expecting her to know her needs and go for them. *She can't always do this! You have to care for her in this way.* You can't always trust that she is speaking her deepest truth, especially in matters of sexuality, *and you must gently challenge her when you feel there is something troubling her.*

Either partner telling the other what they think the other wants to hear is the source of *innumerable* problems in relationship between men and women. If she agrees to do something, but is less than enthusiastic in her agreement, the loving thing to do is to challenge her. It's also in your best interest to challenge her when she accepts or offers to do something, but you aren't getting a strong "Yes" from her. You can talk about it, and the two of you may still decide to do it – trying new things and stretching yours and hers sexual boundaries is good – but you *must* make sure that her ambivalence is being voiced and truly honored. The wise, and maybe loving thing to do, is to do nothing while there is still any trace of her ambivalence.

Women's over-pleasing often comes up around men's requests and women's offers of blow-jobs and anal intercourse. Here is the lesson in that: It's nice when a woman wants to give you a blow-job. Some women enjoy it. Likewise anal play or anal intercourse. Some like it, some do not. For those that do, use lots of lubricant, be slow, and be gentle. But you have to be certain – very certain – that the blow job or ass fuck is "coming from her surplus," meaning that she is so sexually fulfilled that she wants to give to you. ***When her offer is authentic, you can be delighted to accept. When it's not authentic, you will both pay.***

It's also fine to ask for a blow-job, or a fuck, or a fantasy role-play, or whatever it is that turns you on. But back off at the slightest resistance. You would then either need to let go of it entirely, or else renegotiate with her in the spirit of *"what can I do for you that will make this fun for you and worth your while."* Likewise, do not ever treat her sexing with you as a marital obligation of any kind. She is likely to receive that as whoring for pay, which will kill her turn-on and, eventually, your relationship. In every event, ***you would be wise to meet resistance with redoubled attention on her.***

I remember another of my mentors, Justin Sterling, saying, *"Married men forget that they still need to pay for sex."* Words to the wise. You *"pay for sex"* by giving her the attention and appreciation that she desires, including sensual attention. And the gratification, pleasure and gratitude she will return will make you feel like a million dollars.

# 30 The Do-Date Technique of Clitoral Massage [Victor Baranco]

*"Nymphomania represents the breaking through of female sexualit*
*through all the barriers of morality and pretense." – Dieter Duhm*

Victor Baranco's **Do-Date Technique** is a proven way to bring a woma
to orgasm, and will work with most women, even ones who are non-
orgasmic through other methods. This chapter will tell you how. Do-
Dates are not intended to substitute for other types of sexual activity,
but are often an excellent way to begin sexing, or in a first sexual
encounter.

### First thing: take your penis out of the game – for now

This may be a shocking idea to some men. Men want to have sexual
intercourse. That is just fine and you will. ***But only about 25% of women***
***will come through sexual intercourse alone.*** If sexual intercourse is you
obsession, you will lose most women. And things won't go well between
the two of you, whether or not she says anything in the moment. She will
unhappy and she will be afraid to tell you why, even if she knows – and sh
may not know.

*Here is a Golden Rule:* For most women, you should only penetrate her
when one of the following is true:

- She has already come through
  manual or oral stimulation of the
  clitoris. This is the perfect time
  to penetrate her. In fact, for many
  women, sexual intercourse may
  actually be **de-tumescing.** It will
  take them *down* in excitement,
  not up, which is why it is perfect

  > **"TUMESCENCE"**
  >
  > *Refers to the amount of blood-*
  > *flow and lubrication to a woman's*
  > *clitoris, vagina and entroitus (or*
  > *vaginal opening).  It is a good*
  > *indicator of her degree of arousal.*

  to penetrate her after she has already come. She may be soft and
  loving and enjoy everything you do. It's possible she will even come
  again, which would be perfect, but even if not, it probably will be ve

satisfying to her. Most woman do want the experience of penetration, they just don't want it as the beginning of love-making or as the main event in love-making.

- She is already highly aroused and likely to come shortly after penetration. Maybe she will ask you to come inside her. Even if she does ask you, you can still take your time and there will likely be no loss.

- She is one of the minority of women who comes easily in intercourse.

- You are practicing sacred sexuality and are attempting ejaculation control.

***Focus on her and her pleasure first.*** Your pleasure will lose nothing for the waiting. Doubly so the morning after, when she tells you that you are the best lover she ever had and she wants you to do it every day.

## The Do-Date: your basic sexual practice

The **Do-Date** technique is simple. But despite its natural simplicity, most people do not practice it, or they try and substitute other techniques that may not be as effective.

A Do-date begins with communication. It is not fundamentally different from what you would normally be doing with a woman: appreciating her, and communicating / negotiating.

Let's say you are in bed with her, ideally in the initial stage of a sexual encounter that you have been talking about and fantasizing about for days. You have had a conversation – a negotiation – in which you have asked her what she likes in bed, and you have told her what you like. You have perhaps even shared some of your sexual fantasies, if you dare to.

Start by appreciating her beauty and telling her how attracted you are to her. You might gently kiss her and squeeze her or run your hands all over her body. Fondle and pinch her breasts, if you think she will like it: When in doubt, always ask. Ask her to show you how she likes to be kissed – it may be quite different from your style, but you will likely find her style satisfying as well. It's hard to go wrong in these things. *The key words are negotiation, communication and deliberateness,* and their absence is the reason that love acts fail. ***If you simply take on your love-making and your woman's pleasure with more deliberateness, you are likely to become a rock star to her.***

So let's assume that this is going well. You are appreciating her, kissing and fondling her, maybe even talking dirty to her. Enjoy yourself, and be sure to take your time. Let's hope she is starting to respond to you. There will come a point when she will be ready. You will know it. This is the time to ask her if she would like you to touch her clitoris.

If she agrees (and if she does not, just continue what you are doing and ask her again later, or another day), you may lubricate your hand and finger (coconut oil works well since you can also eat it, but Vaseline or water-based sex lubricant is fine too) and spread it over the opening to the vagina leading up to her clitoris. Take the time to be sure you know where her clitoris actually is (hint: ask her), but don't touch it immediately, except maybe briefly. Just move your hand all around in the general area. Stroke her and give her a light massage. Don't put your finger inside her unless she is already quite aroused. You may ask if it's OK to put your finger in her, but be sure you pay attention to her response – "No" or "Not yet" means exactly that.

Talk to her, and also *"feel into her."* Men sometimes feel hurt or put-down by a woman's sexual feedback. But the deliberate lover treasures whatever feedback he receives – it is certain to be excellent information straight from the expert source. She may give you non-verbal feedback, which is as important as words. This includes sounds, breathing rate changes, eye contact signals, and more. If you are not sure about her response, ask her.

In the heat of the moment it may be best to ask her simple Yes or No questions: *"Would you like my finger inside you?"* or *"Would you like more pressure?"* or *"Do I need to move a bit higher?"* Saying *"Tell me what to do now"* is not the best question, especially if she is already responding to you. Ask yes/no questions, or give her a menu: *"I can rub on your clit now or I can just keep on moving around here, what would you like?"* Questions that might require thinking should have been part of your pre-sexing negotiation. In case there has not been a negotiation, for example you are with a new woman and passion has overwhelmed you both, then try and be even more attuned to non-verbals.

When she agrees that you may move on to her clitoris, and not before, you can begin by lightly – very lightly – stroking her clitoris with lubricant. Move your finger up and down and all around. The feeling is quite pleasurable– if you are enjoying yourself, chances are good that she is too. Keep on talking to her – give her feedback about her physical response to you and of your sensations: *"Oh my, your clit got real hard all of a sudden," "this feels really good to me," "oh this really turns me on."* Noises are good too – do and say whatever turns you on as you are pleasuring her. It will likely turn her on too.

It's very likely that after some minutes of manual clitoral stimulation that she will start responding to you – possibly heavily. This is your goal. She may say to you, *"If you continue doing that I will come."* At this point you may relax, because once she starts responding heavily to you, you know you are doing something right. And you are already ahead of 50% of men. So from that relaxation you may be experiencing, feel into her even more. Communicate your relaxation and turn-on to her non-verbally; in other words, use it to increase your attention and connection to her. Imagine thanking her internally for it, and send her that energy. **Making love to a woman is an energy exchange.**

If and when she starts responding heavily to you, the best strategy is to keep on doing what you are doing. Steady-on. Don't change anything, except slightly and as per your instinct or her direction.

Her arousal will come in waves. She will be going up and down, she may experience contractions which will look like she is actually coming, even though she may just be having what's called a "high peak." You can pull back or give more pressure – be guided by your instinct and if in doubt ask her yes/no questions. You can tease her – rather than stroking the clitoris directly, run your fingers in a circle or arc around it for a few strokes. Then come back to the clitoris, and her arousal will rise. Keep on going as long as you can, or as long as it's fun, but usually no less than 15-20 minutes or until she has come at least once.

After several high peaks, or if it looks like she is going down, you can ask her if she has come, as it is often not possible for the partner to distinguish an orgasm from a high peak. Nor should you confuse female ejaculation with female orgasm. Even among women who squirt easily, the orgasm doesn't necessarily occur at the same time. If she hasn't come yet, just continue stimulating her and be open to her direction.

You may want to tell her that you have all the time in the world and she can take as long as she wants. There is no goal to be achieved and you simply want to explore her sexual response and your mutual pleasure.

You will generally *not* want to stop stimulating her until she has come through manual stimulation, one or more times. Unless, of course, she asks you to stop, or asks for something different. The reason is that if you leave her with nothing but high peaks she may feel tense and frustrated afterwards. When in doubt ask her where she is at, because you really can't know whether she has come or not. If she has a high peak and is starting to go down, you might confirm that with her, then back off to kissing and fondling for a while, and wait for her to come up again – if that is what she wants.

All of this is an art, and it cannot be fully taught in a book. Even so, it is possible to have brilliant results simply by being open to her and to her feedback, and by feeling into her as best you can, even if you don't have a lot of sexual experience. *Don't over-think it. Let your finger do what it enjoys. Be guided by your own pleasure and turn-on, in addition to hers.*

### After she comes...

After she comes, you may want to move on to the next stage of the sexual encounter. It is possible, at that point, that she will be willing to do almost anything you want. You can ask for sexual intercourse, or whatever. Alternatively, let her propose or suggest something. She will likely want to reciprocate in some way.

Some women will shut down sexually after coming. She may not even want you to touch her anymore. This could have any number of causes, and it may be quite difficult for you. You may be disappointed and wish that you had just fucked her, but that would have made the situation worse. You will need to negotiate, probably afterwards. Be patient and be kind, she is doing the best she can.

At the end of your love-making, you might try putting your hand over her entire crotch and pressing down firmly. It may bring her down (de-tumesce her) in a way that will be calming and nurturing for her. Try and be there for her – don't just roll over and fall asleep. It is likely that she will want to be held by you, feel her emotional connection to you and her love for you that will have been released by her orgasm. Tell her how much you love her and want her, or just communicate it non-verbally. This is called **post-coital glow** and is very pleasurable – take your time and enjoy it.

You will also probably want to, if not immediately then later, debrief the experience. Find out what each of you liked best, and what you did (or did not do) that might go better next time. This is actually an aspect of foreplay – it prepares you for your next sexual encounter, and will increase the expectation and turn-on for what may happen next.

### What if she is <u>not</u> responding to manual stimulation?

When a woman does not respond to manual stimulation, there could be several reasons.

The first reason is that she is not yet fully comfortable with you or feels some pressure to perform. You would solve the first problem by returning to negotiation and taking your time, and the second by assuring her that you are in no hurry, that all you want is her pleasure and to take care of her, and that however she responds is fine for you – whether she comes or not. If it's your first time being sexual with her and she doesn't come, that is not unusual and nothing to worry about. In fact you may find it wise to approach your first sexual encounter as a **research date**. This means (and you can put it to her explicitly) to play with her so you can learn her sexual appetites and response patterns, with no goal to be achieved, and if orgasm and intercourse does not happen that is fine. In other words, treat your encounter as research toward maximizing hers and your pleasure. Try different things and see what works.

The second reason could be that she is unused to this approach. It's possible that she usually comes with a vibrator, for example. Ask her how she normally comes and then do it with her, or suggest that she do it herself while you watch. Vibrators can be a helpful love-making tool, and can contribute variety and fun. Most vibrators are too intense to be applied directly to the clitoris, but you can put your fingers or hand on her clit and lay the vibrator on top, and she will likely be very happy.

A third possible reason she is not responding is that she is untrained in making herself come. Discuss this with her, and perhaps look for a class or workshop on this. You can encourage her to masturbate and to educate herself on ways to pleasure herself sensually. You can also offer to help her by being her **sexual research partner** (see below). Proposing a Do-Date to a woman you are dating may pique her interest and generate a good conversation even if she says No. Most women appreciate a man being sexually explicit, in a respectful way, early on in the relationship. And many of them actually love it.

## A Variation: the Sexual Research Do-Date

The do-date technique described above can be used with any woman you are dating or are lovers with, especially when the two of you are seeking a relationship. There is a variation of this technique called a **Sexual Research Date** which doesn't necessarily imply, or require, an ongoing relationship.

A **Sexual Research Date** is a negotiated sexual encounter, of fixed duration (usually between 15 and 30 minutes), whose only goal is the exploration of sensation and of sexual pleasure. Some people call this **Orgasmic Meditation (OM)**, a technique created and made popular by Nicole Daedone, although there are a few distinctions between Orgasmic Meditation and Baranco's Do-Date.

The main difference between a sexual research do-date and the regular do-date is that the woman only takes off enough clothing to expose her crotch, and there is no sexual contact except for hand-on-crotch – i.e. there is no kissing, breast-fondling, etc. The man sits or straddles beside her, in the way most comfortable for both, but usually with one leg under and the other leg over the woman. One hand goes under the woman's buttocks, with the thumb resting lightly on the vaginal opening, while the other hand strokes the clitoris with the index finger or middle finger. The difference between an OM and Baranco's Do-Date is the degree of communication – in an OM there is a restricted set of communication, with the focus being on both partners feeling what is happening and detaching from their internal dialogue. The goal is to maximize sensation, not necessarily orgasm. The woman can make requests *("move a bit to the right")* and the man can make offers.

To learn this technique, and understand the numerous benefits, get Nicole's video or attend one of her events, particularly the **TurnOn events** which you can find in many cities and on Meetup.com.

## What's in it for you: the real goal of sex

As a man, you may wonder: what's in it for me in making a woman com through manual clitoral stimulation? When do I get mine?

This is a natural feeling, but here is the thing. *The best way to approach sexuality, the way that has been proven to create the most satisfying results for everyone, is to **approach sexing as a gift.*** A woman who is sexually fulfilled naturally wants to please you and give back to you. ***You want your feminine partner to please you because it gives her pleasure and turns her on, rather than having her please you because she wants you to love her, approve of her or even marry her.*** *This is a critical distinction and is not necessarily binary* – it may be a bit of both. However, a woman who has lost touch with her own pleasure is not in her power and will not serve you well. As a masculine partner, part of your job is to ensure that she maintains focus on her pleasure first – more than on yours. Your pleasure will ultimately come from her sexual fulfillment, and her pleasure from your turn-on as she gives back to you – but her pleasure needs to come first. Decades of research have shown that this works best.

Men are biologically driven to fuck, but they need to re-channel that drive if they wish to have successful relationships. *"Rechanneling"* does not mean to give up the desire to fuck – that would not be healthy (or even possible) – but it does require that we put that biological drive into the context of the larger purpose of sex. Sex is *both* a kind of biological imperative for men, and a tool for connection, transformation and manifestation. All these needs can be fully served, if we pull back, discipline our biological drive, and exercise patience and discernment. We also need to make sure our women are served by the encounter, which is a communication issue. Men need to lead in communication in sexuality even more than other areas.

In all of the higher forms of sex, including sacred sexuality, orgasm is not the goal – not even simultaneous orgasm, although that can be extremely pleasurable. In fact, in most forms of **Tantric sexuality**, men's orgasm can be withheld indefinitely, and sexual energy channeled into higher energy centers and circulated throughout the body. This practice can give men a lot of sexual power, including the ability to have intercourse longer and more frequently, and increase physical vitality. But even in the case of ordinary, or non-sacred, sexuality, it is generally a mistake to push for orgasm or to consider orgasm as the goal of sex. Go for connection, self-awareness and awareness of your partner, and let the orgasm happen by itself – or not. You will be amazed by the amount of fun you can have.

## In conclusion

The basic Do-Date technique *will* get you there with most women. Of course, making love to a woman can be an infinitely rich and complex experience. I am suggesting that you start with solid, deliberate hand-work, or tongue-work, before you try to go to the moon with her. You will likely not go wrong, and you may be ahead of most of the other lovers she has had. *And you will get better every time you play this game with her, as you learn what she likes and as she trusts you more, enabling her to open to you and ask for what she wants.*

A Do-Date is an especially good idea in the early stages of a relationship. She may think that you only want to fuck her, like all her previous boyfriends perhaps. If so, it is easy for you to demonstrate your commitment to her pleasure, and yours will lose nothing for waiting. You might begin by offering her a **sexual research date.**

If you master the basic Do-Date technique you will be off to an excellent beginning. You will be ahead of most men.

And after that, keep on exploring. There is no limit to how high you can go. Playing this game well could be the doorway to your spiritual awakening – and perhaps the only chance you will get for a spiritual awakening in this lifetime.

We have been calling this the **Man/Woman game**, but it is a lot more than a game. It moves up rapidly to engage the deepest (best and worst) parts of both players. It will utterly transform you both. Your friends and family will wonder what happened to you. Don't be afraid to tell them.

# 31 Sexual Variations, Games, and Fetishes

*"Instinctively men have sensed and feared the superior strength of female sexuality." – Dieter Duhm*

Here are a few variations of the basic practice. They are all good. These include:

- Oral sex;

- Sexual positions;

- The 69 position;

- Sexual role play.

**Oral sex** – licking her clitoris. Many women love oral sex. The problem is that your tongue might get tired – you won't have the same staying power as your sturdy forefinger does. Also, you don't have the same *aim* as your finger – you will feel her clit with your finger but your tongue may be off, so she will need to tell you or else you will need the lights on. Also, she may come in a rush before her general sensuality has had a chance to heat up. You'll both have more fun if you can draw it out, 15 to 20 minutes is a useful mark, though of course it is up to her. What you might try, if she really loves oral sex, is to switch back and forth between oral sex and manual stimulation. Many women find that works rather well.

A point here: **Vaginal smell.** Some men find it enticingly delicious, but not all men enjoy oral sex or the smell of a woman's vagina. If that is your situation, you don't have to fight it. It's good to try, but if you are not enjoying it, it's best to retreat to the hand most of the time.

**Sexual positions.** Some positions allow you to manually stimulate her during penetration, some positions don't. There are several helpful, low-stress penetration-plus-fondling positions that you can maintain for a long time without tiring: doggie-style, the cross, and the similar scissors. In any of these positions you can be stimulating her clitoris and fucking her at the same time. In the cross and scissors position, she lies on her back with her knees raised while he lies crossways on his side, now adjust all four legs for comfort and ease – Google these positions for helpful diagrams. Relaxed experimentation with positions can give both players the best of both worlds, provided you both be comfortable. A hanging sex-sling also can be helpful here – she can utterly relax while he stands between her legs to penetrate and fondle her.

**The 69 position.** You will lie head-to-toe with her where you can stimulate her both orally and manually while she sucks on your penis. Many women enjoy having a man's penis in their mouth. And of course this will increase your turn-on too. Many lovers find 69 to be a marvelous position.

**Sexual role play, costumes, BDSM.** Ask her if she would enjoy being lightly tied while you kiss and fondle her. Ask her about scenes of any kind – doctor/patient, daddy/little, flogging, abduction, even rape. Ask her to try different sexual positions and Tantra practices such as Yab/Yum breathing or energy circulation. There is an infinite amount of fun you can have in this arena. Setting the scene by negotiating in advance and preparing the space can be helpful as well as super-fun. The more far-out you and she want to go sexually, the more important is the negotiation.

*All sexual fantasies between consenting adults are good* – even fantasies which, if acted out for real – for example rape or daddy/daughter sex – would be profoundly immoral and probably illegal. Be imaginative and free, but also be careful and be ethical.

And you can always return to the basic Do-Date. It requires little advance negotiation or preparation and will, in most cases, make you a great lover right from the start.

# 32 Negotiating Sexual Differences: Sexual Chemistry and Problems of Desire

*"Like spiritual energy, sexual energy has a cosmic origin." – Dieter Duhm*

Sexual differences – differences in sexual appetite, lack of **Sexual Chemistry,** fetishes that are not shared, communication style mismatches – they all happen. There is, unfortunately, no formula for dealing with these, except to communicate and negotiate.

Many sexual differences can be handled through negotiation, even problems of sexual attraction and Sexual Chemistry. Many women will become attracted to a man they are intimate with, regardless of what he looks like, and many men will become attracted to a woman they are sexual with, even if attraction was not originally present. *The whole question of sexual attraction or "chemistry" is not nearly as big a deal as most people make of it.* Indeed, the obsessive pursuit of chemistry in a relationship, as is common in Internet dating, is a dreary business in which you are liable to lose. I am not saying that chemistry it not important – it is. I am saying that **chemistry is created, you can co-create it.** If you want more chemistry with your partner, get to work: Put your attention on her, learn what she likes, and then do it for her. Chemistry will likely happen.

It's also possible that you are extremely attracted to a woman emotionally and intellectually but Sexual Chemistry is just not there, no matter how much you work at it. In that case, consider negotiating alternative sexual arrangements such as polyamory. Many people argue that mating for life is not the natural human experience. Polyamory is tricky to get right, but there are some good books on the topic[11] and many people do succeed. If you know upfront that you are polyamorous, you will need to state it upfront, as well. Or as soon as practical when beginning a new relationship.

---

11  More Than Two: A practical guide to ethical polyamory, by Franklin Veaux

# 33 Sacred Sexuality and the Stages of Relationship [Chris Menné]

*"Unless and until you access the conscious frequency of presence, all relationships and in particular intimate relationships are deeply flawed and ultimately dysfunctional." – Eckhart Tolle*

## What is Sacred Sexuality?

**Sacred Sexuality** denotes a wide range of practice and beliefs designed to access what Tolle calls *"the conscious frequency of presence"* during love-making. It is sometimes referred to as "Tantric sexuality," although Tantra is not a single or homogenous belief system. Technically, Tantra is a set of ancient spiritual traditions from India, China, and Tibet which share the belief that all of life can be used as the fuel for our awakening. Tantric traditions, which are often not even mostly about sex, explicitly renounce the idea, common in most forms of Eastern spirituality, that to achieve a permanent awakening we must withdraw from the world, relationship attachments, and sex.

---

**CHRIS MENNÉ**

*Chris Menné is an American author, coach and sexual educator. He was an airline pilot for 20 years while he pursued ever deeper studies into spirituality and mysticism. In 2007, at a retreat in India, he experienced a "near-complete dissolution of ego" – a state which he doesn't necessarily recommend for everyone. He then met a woman there, Anya, who was having a similar experience. They shared a powerful state of unity with each other that lasted for weeks. When they returned to the States, they became partners, but the grind of life and career reasons caused them to separate. Chris and Anya now work with conscious singles and couples who want to expand their sexuality into the spiritual realm.*

---

*This is good news to Westerners,* because most of us don't have either the means or the desire to renounce the world in order to awaken to higher consciousness, nor do we want to give up sex. If you desire a spiritual awakening in this lifetime, but don't want to give up sex, then Sacred Sexuality is for you.

*To access the conscious frequency of presence,"* in a relationship means to relate to yourself and your partner as an embodiment, or a manifestation, of a larger entity or presence. It means to accept the fundamental unity that exists between you and your partner at a spiritual level, and to understand that you are far, far larger and more complex than your ego or small self – even, and especially that self who has needs and wants. When you live from the *"conscious frequency of presence,"* your needs and wants may still be there, but they will fade into insignificance in comparison to the power and glory of the larger consciousness or presence of which you are a part. You may feel that larger consciousness keenly, and you may be utterly transformed by that experience. This is the place from which you practice, or attempt to practice, **Sacred Sexuality.**

Now, you don't need to have sex to experience this state of **Presence** or **Being**. However, sex and Being can be extremely synergistic, utterly and profoundly transformational. Sacred Sexuality can be deeply fulfilling at a personal level, energizing and awakening and connecting you to the ultimate source of meaning and of love in the universe. ***It may, indeed, be the best chance that you have to a real spiritual awakening in this lifetime.*** And it is free, and usually a lot of fun, even though the goal is not "fun" exactly, the goal is awakening.

There is absolutely no reason not to try it, and every reason to do so, provided you have a partner whom you trust and who is willing. You do need to have a partner to practice Sacred Sexuality. Of course you can educate yourself on your own, while you are waiting to manifest that partner. You can work on your **Presence** outside of sex.

Many of the ideas in this chapter derive from Chris Menné and his wonderful free ebook that you can get for free on his site SexLoveandPower.com. The most popular modern master of sacred sexuality, however, is David Deida. I will start with a summary of Chris Menné's ideas because some of them are more distinguished than Deida's, especially in terms of the stages of relationship.

### The Stages of Relationship [Chris Menné]

Menné has identified four stages of relationship. The first three are mirrored in Deida's famous **Stages of Relationship.**

While Sacred Sexuality *might* put you into a state of being or awakening most of the time, this is not going to happen for most people. Most of us will be flowing back and forth between the different stages of relationship at different times.

### Stage 1 relationship: Me-Centered and Co-Dependent

- Basis for connection: Agreement and security. Maintain group beliefs.

- Social orientation: Traditional.

- Orientation to awakening from mainstream consciousness: Asleep alone.

- David Deida stage: "Macho jerk / submissive housewife" stage 1.

In this stage, sex is simply an exchange of power between people, within prescribed social roles. There may be dominant and submissive factors. It is essentially "what's in it for me" for both partners. There is little true intimacy, although there can be love. It is mostly about security, predictability, and cultural norms.

### Stage 2 relationship: We-Centered Co-Independent

- Basis for connection: Perceived Value, Enhance the Status Quo, and Compromise.

- Social Orientation: Modern.

- Orientation to awakening from mainstream consciousness: Asleep Together.

- David Deida: "Sensitive wimp" stage 2.

Stage 2 relationships are based on **needs communication and negotiations.** Deida terms stage 2 relationships the "sensitive wimp stage," defining it as equal expectations for men and women (no sexual polarity, or acknowledgement of gender differences). Deida's terminology occurs as dismissive. *If most people in the world could achieve a stage 2 – or perhaps a "high stage 2" such as described in this book, which acknowledges sexual polarity while emphasizing the importance of needs negotiation – then people and our planet would be transformed overnight.*

It is common, incidentally, among practitioners and teachers of Tantric sexuality, to minimize or dismiss early stages of relationship in favor of the higher stages. This is sometimes referred to as "spiritual bypassing." Deida likes to be provocative, and these ideas are inherently provocative. And of course there are always multiple ways of understanding relationships. Indeed, Stage 2 relationships can be on a scale. The important point is that Stage 2 relationship are based on needs negotiation, a distinction that disappears in the higher stages.

## Stage 3: Being-Centered

- Basis for connection: Supporting Internal Alignment. Authentic Connection.

- Social Orientation: Post Modern or New Age.

- Orientation to awakening from mainstream consciousness: Waking-Up Together.

- David Deida: Intimate Communion, or No Boundaries stage 3.

This is the first stage where true **Sacred Sexuality** occurs. This is where the goal of sex is no longer just fun, or even bonding with your partner. You aren't relating to your partner any more as a personality, or as a person with individual needs separate from yours. Needs and personality just fall away and are replaced by something bigger. The goal is awakening, dissolution of ego-boundaries, connection to Being, or to ultimate presence.

## Stage 4: Consciousness, Spiritual, and Source Based.

- Basis for connection: Resonance with One-Another and Universal Truth.

- Social Orientation: Transformative, Contributory, Unifying.

- Orientation to awakening from mainstream consciousness: Waking-Up Together with the Whole.

In stage 4, we go beyond *"waking up together with your lover"* to a global awakening. The boundaries between ourselves and other human beings and even all of manifested reality, dissolve. This is sometimes referred to as "samadhi" – the bliss of divine consciousness. ***Stage 4 is the ultimate desired destination of Sacred Sexuality.***

### Why engage with Sacred Sexuality?

The goal is to dissolve the illusion of our separateness from all other beings and manifested reality, and to get beyond our identification and attachment to our individual body-minds and personalities.

This is a good thing. It could utterly transform how you relate to the world and to other people if you can experience this even briefly. It will, at minimum, make you a deeper and more interesting person. Sexuality could be the most direct path to an experience of awakened living.

Menné writes:

> *"Typically, we see sex as a domain to share love as well as the luscious giving and receiving of sexual pleasure, expressing and building love, and perhaps having children.*
>
> *"But there's much more to sex than that. The sexual drive is a primal force flowing through the fabric of the universe. Without the power behind sexuality, nothing would exist. It's a motivating, driving energy throughout all of existence--and that includes you.*
>
> *"You are not left out of the equation. The Universe did not forget you. In fact, the Universe is now calling to you to remember.*
>
> *"The root of the problem lies in the mundane understandings we've been given of sex and sexual-love. It's an understanding of sex and relationship often based on thoughts, fears, needs, memories, and unexamined ideals.*
>
> *"This is an ego-based understanding... an understanding often cut off from the Universe, and therefore limited.*
>
> *"'Dysfunctional' is a strong term, but we can't say we disagree*

*with Mr. Tolle. Yet, fully grasping what is proposed here involves a significant expansion in consciousness. Many modern approaches to conscious sexuality simply do not address what Tolle is suggesting here. In our work we do.*

*"This is a paradigm shift in human consciousness which is upon us now, and we are being called to inhabit it. And as Tolle suggests, intimate relationships are being particularly impacted by this shift in consciousness when this shift is not addressed. This is a shift beyond our current ego-based understanding of sexual-love.*

*"Simply said, this is a radical shift in perception when it comes to how we experience sex, sexuality, and partnering. And this is a profound."*

Thank you, Chris Menné – beautifully said. Menné is asking us to consider this idea:

**Sexuality is the evolutionary imperative of human reproduction. But it is also, perhaps, the fundamental fuel of the evolution of human consciousness... whether sexual intercourse occurs, or not. Not everyone is aware of this.**

Eckhart Tolle again:

*"On the physical level, you are obviously not whole, nor will you ever be. You are either a man or a woman, which is to say, one half of the whole. On this level, the longing for wholeness – the return to oneness – manifests as male/female attraction, man's need for a woman, woman's need for a man. It is an almost irresistible urge for a union with the opposite energy polarity. The root of this physical urge is a spiritual one: The longing for an end to duality, a return to the state of wholeness. Sexual union is the closest you can get to this state on the physical level. This is why it is the most deeply satisfying experience the physical realm can offer."*

Now, assuming all this is true, let me ask you this:

*Is there anything that you could do, anything at all, that could be of higher value than this?*

*Especially when you consider that it is free, requiring only a momentary surrender to being and/or to your partner, and might allow you to play a key role in the evolution of human consciousness and the healing of the world?*

This global consciousness shift is happening right now, worldwide, inspired by new models of intimacy and human sexuality. This global consciousness shift is beginning now in the bedrooms of America and over the entire world. *I believe it can no longer be stopped, and that it will transform the world as we know it.*

## Spiritual Materialism and Spiritual Bypassing

One of the greatest dangers of all spiritual disciplines is delusion, also known as ego-inflation. It is when we think and believe we are enlightened, but we are actually just using our spiritual training and skills in the service of our egos, or limited body-mind identifications. There are two specific manifestations of this. *All of us – repeat, all of us suffer from these delusions, at times, on the spiritual path.*

> ### SWAMI RUDRANANDA (1928 – 1973)
>
> *Swami Rudrananda, or "Rudi" (born Albert Rudolph) was an American Jewish spiritual teacher, Kundalini Tantra master, and entrepreneur. He was an authentic spiritual genius, achieving high levels of realization while never losing his down-to-earth flair, directness and humor. Rudi ran an Asian art import business in New York City all of his life, believing that a spiritual teacher should not be dependent on his students for his life support. See if you can find a beautiful, out-of-print book by John Mann called* **RUDI: 14 YEARS WITH MY TEACHER.**

**Spiritual Materialism** [Chogyam Trungpa] is when we use our spiritual skill, experience, or knowledge to bolster our egotistic self-concept and to create separation from others. We may lose empathy for other people because we may think, *"What's the matter with these people? They have only to meditate as much as I do and their problems will be solved (and maybe they will get off my back as well, or stop causing me problems)."* **Spiritual Materialism** is an egotistic and arrogant belief system fueled, ironically, by our inaccurate assessment of our own level of spiritual development. *Many great teachers have fallen prey to Spiritual Materialism.*

The cure (often involuntary) to spiritual materialism is to understand that *"the true test of your spiritual success is the happiness of the people around you"* [Swami Rudrananda]. Your spiritual awakening should not put you beyond compassion for others nor beyond a humble attitude. *The extent to which people still trigger you, is the extent to which your work is not done.*

**Spiritual Bypassing** is when we minimize, ignore or attempt to transcend problems or issues that are occurring at lower stages of development, focusing all of our energy and attention on practices relating to higher levels of development, in the hope that the lower-level problems will simply go away.

**Spiritual Bypassing** happens quite often in Stage 2 / Stage 3 conflicts. We may desire to experience a merging with our partner, a dissolution of boundaries. We may even have experienced this state with them, and it was so blissful that we seek only to go back there, desperately. But we can't, maybe because we are upset with them over something they have said or done. Typically, we will blame either ourselves or them for our failure to get over the issue. We may also pretend, to ourselves and to others, that we have overcome the issue. But we haven't. We are, essentially, lying. We are lying in the name of spirituality – again. How humbling.

Some of the communication tools described in Part 7 of this book can be valuable and powerful for resolving Stage 2 / Stage 3 issues relating to Spiritual Bypassing. *These tools work so well because you can only transcend problems at lower levels of development up to a point.* Sometimes, you just have to do your work, put in your time, work directly on the issue in the place it presents. Dissolution of ego-boundaries and the true experience of being is always a gift, an act of grace. If you are not experiencing it, it's because your work at a certain stage or level of development is not done. *Stop arguing with God, or feeling bad for your failures, and do the work.*

### What's next?

Let's assume that you are now persuaded of the benefits of **Sacred Sexuality.** You want to try it. What do you actually do?

Unfortunately, there is no formula for achieving these states, no set of steps and actions that will predictably get you to the goal. There is also no fairness in achieving these states, in that these states are always given to you by grace, they are not something that you earn through your work. You can practice for years and get nowhere, or you can talk to your partner tonight, try something different with her, and be transported in a moment into an experience of pure being, an experience that you won't forget for the rest of your life.

In fact, people often have profound experiences quite early on in their practice, experiences that don't repeat and that they then spend years trying to recapture. But that is the point. It's not about achieving anything. It's about "being," which means to accept what is. There is a good reason that God does what he does. You cannot understand this, from your limited perspective.

Nevertheless, there are many helpful practices. You have to begin somewhere. As you begin this journey, which could be the single most important journey of your life, be aware of the following:

- First, that Sacred Sexuality is a subset of ordinary spirituality. In other words, practices like prayer, meditation, yoga, spiritual reading, exercise and healthy lifestyle, even positive thinking and stage 2 intimacy – besides just being a humble, kind and loving person – might be important to get you there.

- And second, the strength of your intention might be *the* determining factor. *"Love is an intention"* [Jerry Jud]. *"Faith as small as a mustard seed"* [Jesus]. *"Pray for the willingness to have your shortcomings removed"* [Alcoholics Anonymous].

# PART 6: THE MAN/WOMAN GAME IN CULTURE AND PHILOSOPHY

The cultural and philosophical context of the **Man/Woman** game. This section covers philosophical topics that don't fit within the "love manual" that is the heart of this book.

# 34 The Inner Game of Masculine and Feminine [Shirley Luthman]

*A true leader is when the people say, after the work is done: "We did it ourselves." – Lao-Tzu*

## Shirley Luthman's basic idea

Psychologist and therapist Shirley Luthman wrote two seminal books, **INTIMACY: THE ESSENCE OF MALE AND FEMALE** (1977) and **COLLECTION: A CONTINUATION OF INTIMACY** (1980). These books, and particularly **COLLECTION**, cover the optimal relationship of masculine and feminine forces within an individual, and they also have some profound insights on the power of, and also limitations of **Structures.** A Structure is a developmental system or model, such as I'm presenting in this book.

These books are out of print. You may be able to pick up a used copy on line. **COLLECTION** is a powerful book if you can get your hands on it, so let's begin with a summary of Luthman's views on masculine/feminine.

> ### SHIRLEY LUTHMAN (1929 – 2011)
>
> *Luthman was a psychologist and therapist. She lived most of her life in the San Francisco Bay area where she taught, practiced psychology and wrote. She made important contribution to the field of family therapy and is the author of many books, including **COLLECTION: A CONTINUATION OF INTIMACY** that is one of my primary sources. Luthman's ability to see the truth in people and her unfailing generosity touched many lives. She believed that the real foundation for human transformation was the laboratory of her own interactions. She ran her life as an ongoing experiment in learning and teaching love, modeled the ideas in her books (effortless manifestation), and she guided many people in this journey.*

Luthman's books deal with Sexual Polarity as the internal relationship between masculine and feminine forces inside the individual. Here the **masculine** elements refers to the aspects that are active, rational, single-pointed consciousness and production-driven, while the **feminine** aspects are receptive, intuitive, diffuse consciousness and pleasure-driven. ***When these forces are in correct relationship, the*** *masculine goal and primary source of meaning and fulfillment lies service to the feminine and to its pleasure goals, while the feminine goal and primary source of meaning lies in maximizing its own pleasure and vitality, and by extension the pleasure and vitality of i internal masculine partner.* Each force must be continually giving the other feedback and relating to it. When this is done correctly, the resul is what Luthman calls **Personal Power.**

Luthman and I both believe that playing a sexual polarity game correctly, whether we are playing internally, or externally as in the Ma Woman game, takes us closer to the realm of **Perfect Manifestation** – the highest form of Personal Power. This is when the Universe aligns with you without any effort. It is when you barely have to say the word and it happens.

This is Luthman's basic idea, but she also has some profound insights what she calls "Structures."

### The nature of Structures

**Structures** are developmental models, which are similar to life philosophies, intellectual frameworks, or belief systems designed to support life. They serve as a means of articulating our values and guiding our choices. This book is an example of a Structure, fundamentalist Christianity is a Structure, secular humanism and atheism and even Nazism are Structures. *Structures are essential to life.*

According to Luthman, Structures are useful to the extent that they are a good match between the true nature of reality and a person's inner life or developmental needs. Reality has an infinite number of dimensions and therefore there are, potentially, an infinite number of Structures. The problem, in human terms, is that a person's inner life and developmental needs are continuously expanding. For example, it not at all unusual to go from a fundamentalist Christian, to an atheist c secular humanist viewpoint, to a mystical view of life.

Each of these three Structures served the person on their journey at the right time, helping them along to the next stage of growth and development. Each stage failed at some point, and needed to be replaced or extended. This idea is similar to the principle called **inclu and transcend** within the theory of spiral dynamics [Don Beck and

Chris Cowan], which has been taken up and popularized by philosopher Ken Wilber.

All Structures, to the extent that they are useful, reflect some fundamental truth about the human condition or about an individual's developmental needs. And yet no single Structure can ever fully or permanently model or assist a person's life path, because life is designed to infinitely expand. Life, and love, will outgrow any Structure we try and impose on it. *This is Luthman's second fundamental idea.* It is also exactly what is going on in modern science: Newtonian mechanics to quantum physics to quark theory. We are reaching towards ever higher models, or distinctions, on the nature of reality. Each stage includes and transcends the previous one. This happens inside the individual as well, in our life's journey.

Life's desire to expand – to become more complex and more inter-related – is the fundamental nature of all creation, and of God. *To love well is nothing other than to become more inter-related, which is the same as expansiveness.* Luthman identifies this fundamental desire in each of us to expand as part of the **feminine** and relates it to intuition, arguing that intuition always knows where it wants to take us: expansion into greater pleasure, vitality, and love. And Luthman identifies the Structure, which is the internalized belief system, the thing that guides our actions, as part of the **masculine**.

> ### KEN WILBER (1949 – )
>
> *Wilber is an American writer and philosopher. He is the creator of "Integral Theory" and has written more than 20 books on topics related to spirituality, mysticism, and developmental psychology. As the inventor of Integral Theory and the founder of the Integral Institute in 1999, Wilber has been nicknamed the "Einstein of consciousness." His theories became a sensation in the academic and "spiritual" community after the founding of the Integral Institute, but fizzled out for lack of leadership. There is an excellent article called "The Rise and Fall of Ken Wilber" by Mark Manson that explains what happened. It is a good story, a story in many ways of self-deception or ego-inflation. Google it. Wilber's autobiographical* **GRIT AND GRACE** *is a deeply moving story of love and awakening, about his wife who died of cancer. He currently suffers from a rare neurological disease that has severely restricted his creative output in the last decade.*

## Masculine responds to feminine – whether it is aware of it or not

So what happens in healthy human development is that our "intuition," also known as the feminine force that primarily seeks and values *pleasure and love,* calls on the masculine force that seeks and values *production and assertion.* In other words, in an ideal developmental scenario, *the masculine forces inside the individual serve and respond to the feminine.*

*Neither force can be complete without the other:* masculine is incomplete and meaningless without a feminine to serve, and feminine is incomplete and powerless without a masculine to back it. *"Men without women tend to be flat, predictable and outwardly destructive; women without men tend to be unfocussed, emotionally self-indulgent and inwardly destructive"* [David Deida, paraphrased].

This idea is fundamental. In this book we have been applying Luthman's basic idea to the real-world problem of the ideal relationship between a masculine person and a feminine person. Luthman is referring to *an inner relationship* of masculine and feminine, whereas we have been exploring the *outer relationship* of masculine and feminine people. The natural role of a masculine person – some would say the inevitable or inescapable role, as we are programmed into this by evolution – is to serve women and try to make them happy. *"Women call, men respond"* [Victor Baranco]. Some would even say that men respond to the feminine and to feminine people whether we are aware of this or not. We are doing it all the time, consciously or unconsciously. And in addition to this, all people respond to their own internal feminine. According to Luthman, understanding and supporting the natural internal relationship of masculine and feminine – fundamentally the relationship between pleasure-drives and production-drives, between our desire for happiness and our desire for success – is the key to Personal Power. This internal relationship often goes wrong, however, as will be described next.

## How human development (maturation) really happens

Life evolves. Yesterday's solutions don't necessarily work with today's problems. So here, according to Luthman, is what happens in a best-case scenario of human development:

*We see that our current structure does not work any more. Our internal feminine is clear on that, and creates the intention for something else to come into our life. Our internal masculine hears that request and gets to work on it. Soon enough, some other Structure comes into being, one more suited to our current developmental needs, which then empowers other types of manifestation. And so on.*

But here is what is more likely to happen – and particularly at the beginning stages of your journey to perfect manifestation. One of two things.

- One: the feminine hears the need in the still inner voice but pays it no mind. Or else it disrespects it: *"You can't want THAT, surely, Hush."* or maybe *"I don't deserve that"* or *"Look, things are going well, let's not rock the boat."* So the internal feminine doesn't communicate and the internal masculine goes back to watching football, metaphorically speaking. Nothing happens.

- Or two: the feminine does communicate the need but the masculine doesn't respond, or fails to provide support. It might say: *"You want WHAAAT??? That's crazy."* Or *"I can't do it. Give it up."* Again nothing happens, at least immediately.

## The nature of "healing crises" and of all manifestation

And so the need sits there unfulfilled, until – and this is important – *life itself takes over and creates a crisis,* also known as a "healing crisis," but more commonly known as "shit happens" or "God hit me with a 2x4." Money dries up, the car explodes, relationships go bad, you lose your health, whatever.

And then you sit in your self-pity and loneliness and misery until you are ready to do something about it – or not. And as soon as that happens, as soon as your energy returns, the flow of manifestation resumes, and then you get it: *You realize how much better off you are now than if you had stayed in that old job, kept that old car, continued taking as poor care of yourself as you were doing before, failed to make that important communication, or enforced those boundaries with people.*

So basically, here are your two, and only two practical choices: you can "move shit" fast and voluntarily (aka "personal power"). Or you can do nothing and wait for life to "move shit" for you. The latter takes more time and is emotionally draining and sometimes traumatic. There is a third choice as well: You can stubbornly refuse all feedback (continue as you are) and be killed, or else die internally.

What determines whether you "move shit" quickly or slowly? One thing: *the quality of that internal communication* between masculine and feminine forces inside you. The continuous giving and receiving of feedback. **The willingness to receive negative feedback, and take it to heart, is key.**

The art of receiving negative feedback gracefully and thoughtfully, in either the internal or external relationship, is where almost everyone goes wrong. But whatever the reasons our communications fail, we must truly *respond to the other in order to grow.* Without this, there is no relationship, and without relationship there is no manifestation. There is just an endless stream of healing crises ending, sooner or later, in death.

To summarize, here are your choices according to Luthman: surrender to life's expansion voluntarily, which requires accepting the feedback, and live in joy for the most part; or resist it, and live in suffering for the most part. Either choice eventually takes you to expansion, life is clever in that way. But the first way is a lot faster and more pleasurable, and hence more powerful.

*These are, of course, the exact choices a man faces in the outer game of masculine and feminine:* surrender fully, but within your value system, into your attraction and desire for her, and accept her direction. Or, resist her direction, and then either live without women, or live with an unhappy and angry woman and continue to flounder. It is difficult for a man to be truly successful when his woman is not backing him, or else when he is continually dealing with Dark Feminine drama, added to his own dramas of course.

## What is the value of all this?

It is another way of understanding the **Man/Woman game.** *In human developmental terms, the creation and destruction of Structures, and optimizing the inner game of masculine and feminine, is precisely mirrored in the outer game of masculine and feminine.*

It's brilliant and beautiful. The inner and outer games of masculine and feminine complement and support each other perfectly. You can play this game in any realm, internal or external, and doing so will move you towards the perfect manifestation of effortless success. *"A true leader is when the people say, after the work is done: 'We did it ourselves.'"* [Lao-Tzu].

That is the definition of *"effortless success."* Everybody is doing their best work in perfect harmony: the leaders listen and persuade, the intellectuals think, the workmen dig, the builders build, the salesmen sell. And everyone acknowledges and appreciates the others for their unique and essential contributions, living in flow and in gratitude. You can play this game within yourself, as well, as Luthman teaches. You can end the internal war of sub-personalities. Just call an internal meeting, declare a cease-fire, and commit to never again finding anyone wrong, whether they be real people or your own internal sub-personalities.

***This is the human destiny, the reason we were created, the inevitable path of evolution, the perfect society towards which we are heading.*** There may still be time, before we destroy the planetary ecosystem that sustains us.

## Ah, the ego

Many people talk about the ego as if it were something that needs to be suppressed if we are to reach our final spiritual destination. However, you might consider the ego to be a sub-personality, as in Cheri Huber's view. If you feel your ego is running your life, and you want it to stop, don't imagine that you can fully suppress it, or even quiet it for more than a moment, through exercise, meditation, spiritual practice, or whatever. Instead, acknowledge that if your ego is running the show, it's because "you," representing the union of all your sub-personalities, have not taken leadership yet. **You need to step up and lead,** and you do this by *including* ego and its viewpoints. Ego keeps us alive, what a wonderful thing. Thank him for it, and then give him a seat at the table. Give him the job of managing your survival, while you go out dancing with Shakti and creating the world. It will make him very happy to have a job, and you will feel your home is safe while you are out. It's a win-win.

# 35 Spiritual Underpinnings of Sexual Polarity, and the Future of Love

*"Both halves of the human being, man and woman, have searched for each other for generations and always missed one another"* – Dieter Duhm

*"Enlightenment is when you realize that what was planned was a party"* – Victor Baranco

If you are reading this, you are probably in the top 1% of the world's population in terms of your ability to manifest your dreams and *"contribute to life"* [Marshall Rosenberg]. You are, very probably, well on your way (if such is your desire) to being a *"force of nature,"* as per George Bernard Shaw:

*"This is the true joy in life, being used for a purpose recognized by yourself as a mighty one. Being a force of nature instead of a feverish, selfish little clod of ailments and grievances, complaining that the world will not devote itself to making you happy."*

*"Complaining that the world will not devote itself to making you happy"* describes the fundamental human growth challenge: taking responsibility for the fulfillment of our own needs, also known as **asking for what we want.** *Taking responsibility for our needs does not mean – as our dominant cultural model would teach us – fulfilling our needs by ourselves always.* It means initiating the communications necessary to fill these needs. These communications will be more effective – and reciprocal – when we *accept to look at ourselves throug the eyes of others.*

The reason that I am imagining that you are already a *"force of nature"* simply because you are reading this paragraph, is this: you already are in the 10% of the world's population that has the education and resources to be reading this. And out of those few, maybe 10% are consciously seeking to become more loving. This puts you in the 1% a it's highly probable that if you really take it on, get the support you ne continue educating yourself, and run your life as an ongoing experime in learning and teaching love, that you will achieve whatever you wan in life. *This level of consciousness puts you in the top 1% of people on the planet in terms of manifestation.*

If this is true, think about it. Wow. What a gift. And what a responsibility has been handed to you.

## The Godhead in each of us

By following the path of love, you will be standing with your lover in the crucible of creation, the source of life and of all manifestation, you and your woman as a microcosm of the eternal interplay of masculine and feminine. You will be Shiva, dancing with Shakti and creating the world. How this works is a great mystery, a force beyond words and conceptualization, it is the Godhead in each of us. Indeed, it is the fastest pathway that most of us have available to us for reaching God. Sexuality is the source of a great deal of human creativity, invention, and many wonderful aspects of being human.

## A bold new area of speculation: the future of love

Let's consider now the logical outcome of the state of being that I am describing.

What if it were true that playing in the field of Sexual Polarity was actually the fastest way, for many of us, to happiness and success – these being, respectively, the feminine and masculine goals? And what if "success" might include things such as *power, wealth, and influence?* I mean this in the best sense –the power to impact people's lives in a positive way, as in servant leadership, or the ability to create organizations or platforms that would have a positive impact on the world... such as I myself aspire to, for instance, by writing this book.

And regardless of whether we actually gain wealth and influence, what if all who are playing this game could become *extravagantly and deliriously happy, and sharing that happiness with everyone we meet, and hence extremely attractive to others.* They would want to hang out with us, they would ask us the secret of our happiness and success, **and then they would copy us**. And we would help them, we would teach them how to love and how to be happy... at least to the degree that any individual can be fully happy, in a world where most people continue to suffer and lead limited lives.

And hence, maybe, we could ignite a kind of *cultural virus... a highly contagious one,* and that the number of people playing this game would grow and grow until eventually virtually everyone would be living and loving well. The virus would multiply through our increasingly extended network of relationships, as people would want to model the happiness and success that we would enjoy. A happiness which, unlike the happiness and success enjoyed by the ruling and intellectual classes in previous generations, would be *generous and inclusive and more related to an internal self-generated state than to external wealth or influence...* which would make this state both friendlier to the world's resources, and perhaps accessible to people by the simple means of an *internal decision.*

## The true purpose of Evolution

What if the purpose of evolution – God's purpose – is simply that **we have a good time** (including a lot of great sexual loving, for those so inclined). *"Enlightenment is when you realize that what was planned was a party"* [Victor Baranco].

*And what if this were actually the fulfillment of Jesus's prophecy that "the meek shall inherit the earth"?* I choose to interpret "meek" not so much as being a door-mat, letting other people walk all over me, but as the ability to be present, to listen, to give attention, to take negative feedback calmly and thoughtfully, to choose happiness and love boldly, and to have enough ego-awareness or emotional maturity to consider other people's deep needs *alongside our own* as we go about our daily lives... *while not demanding reciprocity in our care and consideration of others... which Jesus would also be aligned with.*

What if?

Speculation. I am dreaming.

*But it is not my dream alone.*

# PART 7: COMMUNICATION TOOLS AND RESOURCES

New communication tools and practices are going to be essential to your success. Some of these are well-known (Marshall Rosenberg's NON-VIOLENT COMMUNICATION), others have never been published before but are immensely powerful (Withholds, Hexes, and *"You don't need to get what you want if you can express what you want"*).

You will also learn a community-building game called **Hot Seats**, which you can use to build your own community and become a leader in the movement towards a more loving world.

# 36 Non-Violent Communication

*"Your presence is the most precious gift you can give to another human being." – Marshall Rosenberg*

Marshall Rosenberg's Non-Violent Communication (NVC) is, on the surface, a communication model for resolving conflicts between people, but it is much, much more than that. It is an attitude and a set of communication tools designed to evoke, express, and fulfill human needs – and particularly needs for closeness, trust, authenticity, and vulnerability.

It is human nature to criticize your partner and **make them wrong** when they do not meet one of your needs. But you will rapidly learn the foolishness of this approach. What you can do instead is *to learn to speak in the language of feelings and needs* – rather than the language of judgment, criticism, demand and make-wrongs. This is the foundational practice of NVC.

In NVC, any conscious expression of a need to another person is a gift, as it gives them the opportunity to contribute to you and hence make life more wonderful for both of you. This is particularly true when the need is expressed without judgment or demand.  But as you get more skillful in the practice of NVC, you will become able to listen for the feelings and needs underlying all human communications – even communications that are expressed as judgments or demands – and this listening will give you the capacity to give a loving response, a response that may completely defuse the situation and lead to everyone's needs being met. It is an extraordinarily powerful practice, and it is 100% aligned with the relationship model presented in this book.

Note that the NVC perspective on "needs" goes against our entire cultural programming, which is that having needs which we cannot meet for ourselves is somehow sub-optimal, un-evolved or un-spiritual at best, or even shameful – that it makes us a lesser person to be dependent on other people. ***The truth is, we are all inter-dependent.*** None of us can fully meet our needs for ourselves. *"Nobody is healed alone"* [Course in Miracles]. NVC teaches that expressing needs in a way that doesn't come across as a judgment or a demand is a loving thing to do. This requires, however, that we have some awareness of other people and their desire or capacity to help us – in other words, that we accept *"No"* as a valid answer.

The basic formula of NVC is referred to as OFNR for Observation, Feeling, Need, Request. For instance: *"I noticed you have not done last night's dinner dishes yet. I feel annoyed because I value cleanliness, and also because I need the sink to make my dinner. Would you be willing to take care of that before my dinner-time?"*

Using NVC effectively requires a certain attitude and quality of listening even more than formulas or techniques, and this is where beginning students of NVC often go wrong. NVC, when done well, is a profound practice that requires almost a complete re-wiring of our normal patterns of speaking and listening. The fundamental work of NVC is to evoke and discern other people's feelings and needs, and then to mirror them back or express them on their behalf. **Discerning and mirroring other people's needs is one of the greatest acts of love that you can do.**

Expressing your own feelings and needs, without any judgments or demands that the other person meet them, is also a high form of loving. You are giving another person the opportunity to make a difference to you, and to make both yours and their life more wonderful by loving you. And you are also modeling for them how they can get their own needs met. This is the circle of love.

The concept of feelings and needs within NVC, and the practices it encourages, are powerful and profound. If you can, find an NVC class or practice group and take your lover there. It will deepen your relationship for sure, and it could even change your life.

# 37 Withholds

*"...and the greatest Withhold is love." – Victor Baranco*

**Withholds** are an important and powerful emotional communication tool that is still, despite its unusual effectiveness, relatively unknown and unused. I will present here a version of the technique that is derived from Victor Baranco. The practice is also related to psychologist Harville Hendrix's *"Is there more"* exercise, and is fully compatible with NVC, although not officially part of the NVC model.

## What is a Withhold?

A **Withhold** is any emotion or response to another person or to an event that has not yet been expressed. Withholds can be positive or negative. **Positive Withholds** are the failure to appreciate people and tell them how much we care for them, while **Negative Withholds** include the failure to express a feeling or an unmet need.

***Withholds, whether they be positive or negative, kill intimacy.*** Have you ever seen couples who simply don't talk to each other any more? The reason is likely that they have let Withholds accumulate. The more you let Withholds accumulate, the harder it is to communicate anything at all, because any kind of request or negative feedback that you give will start an avalanche of counter-claims and resentments. You will both give up the attempt to share anything important at all, and your relationship will be dead.

Do not let this happen! Clear your Withholds with your partner immediately, in the moment the distressing feeling occurs, whenever possible. In cases where something happens but you are not able to respond immediately, clear it later.

Withholds are a way to clear **Emotional Charge,** which has been defined in Chapter 14. Emotional charge is just raw, unprocessed emotion. "Unprocessed" means that the emotion has not been subjected to a process of discernment. It simply exists in your gut and the fact that you have not said it is creating distance and unsettling you. You know that you will feel better once you have said it, but you can't bring yourself to do it. Maybe you are afraid of hurting your partner or making them angry, or maybe you are ashamed of having the feeling or need in the first place, or you judge it as wrong or "not nice." But you have the feeling, and it won't go away. You are suffering. The inability to express this feeling is making you feel distant from your partner and causing you to shut down emotionally. You have to do something because the situation has become unbearable. You feel the relationship is at stake, if not your sanity. ***What you can do to resolve this situation is to deliver a Withhold.***

Many people are simply overwhelmed by the negative feelings they experience with their intimate partners. They don't even know where to begin, and are afraid of saying anything at all lest it lead to anger or reactivity, and make the situation worse. *But the more you fail to speak your truth, the worse it will become.* Sometimes in relationship, you just have to leap, and trust that things will sort themselves out. The relief you will experience will be in direct proportion to the pain you were feeling before. **Open your heart to your lover.** You may get hurt, or hurt your partner, but most of the time you will both feel better at the end, maybe hugely better. Indeed, you may find this process addictive once you get the hang of it. You may kick yourself that it took you so long to start sharing yourself honestly with another human being – especially the feelings that you think you have no right to have, or that you judge as unkind, selfish or immature.

Fortunately, Withholds are quite easily cleared. The structure makes it safe to say whatever it is you have not yet spoken, and is a fantastic way to begin to resolve the underlying emotional need.

**How to deliver a Withhold**

You say: *"[their name], I have a withhold, are you willing to hear it?"*

They responds: *"Sure,"* or otherwise give you permission to share.

And then you tell it: *"I felt stupid when you said that last thing."* Or whatever.

They end the cycle with a simple, flat *"Thank you,"* and that's it.

A Withhold can be about you, about them, about anything. It can be big or small, life-changing or utterly trivial. You would be wise to avoid assigning blame or shame in your Withholds – in general, try and give the least harsh message that fully communicates the emotion – but you are allowed to say whatever you want. Do not censor the emotion, nor be overly concerned with hurting your partner's feelings or making them angry. They will have an opportunity to respond later, if they choose.

One of the agreements in delivering Withholds is that your partner should only respond with your permission... that is, in the form of another Withhold to you. You would both be wise, however, to let a Withhold sit for a few minutes before responding to it, or else respond at another time. Even more so if the Withhold is big.

If the issue has been going on for some time or you are feeling really triggered, you can ask your partner to **Pull Withholds** from you. You may ask them for 10 to 15 minutes of their time, or longer. If they agree, you would deliver the first Withhold, and your partner would say *"Thank you, is there more?"* This would continue until you are done or until the time is up. Afterwards, you might invite your partner to do the same.

Withholds can be about anything and can be delivered to anybody with whom you have the agreement. You can also deliver them to non-present third-parties or social groups: *"Mom, there is something I've withheld from you,"* or *"Social Security Office, I have a Withhold."* Your partner would then represent the missing person or entity, and respond in the standard way: *"Thank you, is there more?"*

### The agreements to give and receive Withholds

There are two important agreements in giving Withholds.

- First, your partner must explicitly give permission to hear the Withhold. That is why you always ask for permission before delivering a Withhold. If your partner is not available in the moment, they could say so and come back to you later.

- Second, do not consider any Withhold as the truth, or even (and especially) as a mature emotion. This agreement must be in place for the structure to work.

With these agreements in place, both partners may find it immensely freeing to be able to say something to the other with the understanding that it will not be judged, nor even necessarily responded to. Remember a Withhold is in the nature of a raw emotion or a need. When used in the best way, a Withhold communicates an intention to let go of your **emotional charge** around an issue or problem. It is an invitation for collaboration around the need that underlies the emotion. For this reason, giving Withholds is a fantastic way to open a negotiation. It will likely cut in half the time of any negotiation you take on with your partner, if you simply begin by sharing Withholds.

*Withholds can be thought of as an emotion that has been attached to a judgment or belief system.* You deliver the Withhold not sure either of the maturity of the emotion nor of the accuracy of the underlying belief system. When you express a Withhold, you are implicitly stating that what you are saying could be false (i.e. a false belief system) or, at best, not necessarily your truest or deepest feeling on the matter. In essence, you are "trying out" the feeling in order to find your deepest truth, or else to let go of the distressing feeling altogether by putting it out there.

Because you are opening a communication with the assumption and prior agreement that you could be totally wrong, and that what you are about to say is probably entirely your own stuff, your partner may be less defended and more open to you. You are inviting your partner's non-judgmental listening around an emotion or a need that you are experiencing. Together, you might be able to reach clarity on this need soon, and with pleasure. In fact, the process can be pleasurable for both people. Giving and receiving Withholds can be thought of as the purest form of love exchange, because you are trying to let go of your make-wrongs towards your partner, and because you are asking them to help you by listening non-judgmentally and non-reactively. As already stated when you ask someone for help, and are genuinely open to receiving it, you are giving them the opportunity to love you, thereby making both yours and their life more wonderful.

*Fundamentally, a Withhold is a request for attention and collaboration around an emotional issue.* It is possible to resolve a great many emotional issues rapidly in Withholds even before beginning any kind of negotiation. Withholds are a variation of *"you don't need to get what you want if you can express what you want"* (see Chapter 40).

You would both be wise to give Withholds well before the tension on a particular issue rises to the point where a fight is likely to occur. Some couples have pre-set times for sharing or pulling Withholds – once a week, or even every day at an agreed time.

*Withholds are one of the most powerful tools in your communication arsenal. Use them well, and you will preempt many, many problems.*

## Giving Withholds vs. "Sharing Feelings"

The distinction between Withholds and ordinary "sharing of your feelings" is important and easily misunderstood, and worth exploring. It is actually the source of all kinds of problems in communication between people, and especially in communication with women.

Sharing your feelings with another person, say in a normal conversation, can be a beautiful and loving thing to do, a way to connect more deeply. The problem arises when you need to share negative feelings.

According to NVC, negative feelings that you have towards another person are often, and maybe always, related to an unmet need of yours. The issue is that in sharing your raw emotion with them, it is easy to make them wrong. This means it is all too easy to throw in judgments or demands into the communication. *Once the other person feels attacked or blamed, it becomes more difficult for them to hear you and less likely that your need will be met.* It is, unfortunately, human nature to make people wrong when they don't meet our needs – and *it virtually guarantees that they will continue to not meet the need going forward.*

An actual example may help you understand the process. I will analyze this interaction at some depth.

My partner said to me, *"Marc, I feel that you are provoking an argument. Are you aware that you are doing this? Do you know that you do this with women? All you seem to care about is arguing and being right."*

The problem with this communication is that *"provoking arguments"* is her belief of what is happening. This is different than my belief, which is that I am naturally curious about people, their feelings and needs, and that I enjoy getting to an underlying truth about where people are at. Sometimes I like to push those boundaries, attempting some serious probing of their deeper feelings and needs. This can look like provocation.

And so, we are both right. **The fact that she feels that I am "provoking arguments" makes her right by definition, feelings are always true that they reflect a true underlying need.** But still, this communication is NOT likely to get her need met. Rather, it is likely to make me want to argue even more, because she has **made me wrong** – that is, given a judgment that I don't agree with, that comes from a perspective other than mine.

This is sometimes called an *"irresponsible communication"* because it is unlikely to result in any needs being met. We communicate irresponsibly because we haven't done our work of discernment around an unmet need and the feelings that underlie it. We simply dump the feeling, with all the attached make-wrongs, on to the other person.

*In this example her need is for greater empathy from me, with less arrogance.* She is saying that she would like me to listen better, and maybe be less invested in being right. She may also be saying that my style of pushing, or probing, is exhausting for her, and to stop it.

On a good day, I might be able to hear this and acknowledge it, and then change how I am relating to her. I could realize that I am not serving her by holding onto my agenda, and just drop it. But let's say I am having a bad day. I may not *feel* like dropping my agenda. **I may just want to argue with her to "make her wrong for making me wrong."** This is the natural human response to being attacked or made wrong: defend or counter-attack. From here the situation rapidly escalates, leaving everyone feeling angry and unheard, and sowing the seeds for future comebacks on the same issue. The argument can go on for years.

### And this is where Withholds can be useful and powerful

So: a more effective communication, an NVC communication, could go something like this:

*"Marc, I am really not enjoying this conversation or your attitude right now. It feels like you are provoking me. I could be wrong about this, but I want to change the energy of this interaction. Can you hear what I am saying? I need more empathy from you."*

Can you see why this is a much more effective communication than the first one? First, she is stating her deeper feelings and needs rather than waiting for me to imagine or discern them through her make-wrong: *"I am not enjoying this conversation"* is a feeling-statement, one which I cannot really argue with as it's about her rather than me. And second, she is asking for what she wants – empathy – rather than telling me what she doesn't want – provocation.

However, she may not have enough internal clarity to frame and deliver the responsible communication. She may just be angry or frustrated and convinced that I am, indeed, provoking her, and probably deliberately. *Withholds can clean up this mess.*

**If she senses that the argument is going nowhere because she is making me wrong and I am reacting to that, then she could try to give the same communication in a Withhold:** *"Marc, I have a Withhold. Will you hear it?"* And after I agree: *"I feel you are provoking me."*

By this, she is communicating two things:

- First, she is not declaring her feeling as either objectively true (as in a mature emotion), or as the deepest truth in the matter. This reduces my reactivity.

- Second, she is enrolling me in helping her to figure out the underlying need – what am I actually doing that irks her so.

**By putting the matter as a Withhold, she is actually making a much more effective communication.** Of course, it will only work with a person who understands the Withhold communication structure. It is a powerful structure, one which is 100% aligned with NVC, provided that both you and your partner are willing to play.

She may not be willing to play. She may not be able or willing to take that much responsibility for the fulfillment of her own need. I can try gently pointing this out to her, or I can just give her what she wants – empathy – and from that place, I can stop arguing with her.

*It's also possible that I have such poor empathy skills that she gives up trying to initiate any deeper communication with me at all.* She may consider Withholds to be horseshit, because I haven't yet demonstrated the value to her. She may just prefer to "share her feelings" with me in a regular conversation, making me wrong left and right, because it's better than not saying anything at all. She may also just be communicating that she is done with me, or at least done with this particular way I have of relating to her (arrogance). In all these cases, it's a call for greater empathy. Almost all arguments between people, deep down, are a call for greater empathy.

This example is very real to me, and a constant challenge: I can get triggered when I feel people are not listening to me or making me wrong, *but rather than saying so directly, I make clumsy and at times obnoxious attempts to educate them on how I want to be spoken to, with the underlying arrogant attitude that I know how to communicate better than they do.* As such, she is right, I *am* provoking her, because I am coming across as a know-it-all, and I am oblivious to this effect on other people.

***In this instance, I can change the tone of the conversation as easily as she can, simply by acknowledging my unmet need and communicating honestly from that place.*** Either party in a broken communication can set it right and return to a field of love. I can either give empathy, or, alternatively I can give my own Withhold: *"I have a withhold, will you hear it? I am sorry you feel that I am provoking you, but I am feeling now attacked and made wrong by you. I feel frustrated and angry because you are not getting me. I am just trying to understand you so that I can feel closer to you."* And from there, I can start a negotiation with her – figuring out what she and I both really want to hear from the other – a negotiation that will likely go a lot quicker and smoother because, by receiving my Withhold, she has demonstrated a willingness to listen to me. I can relax from trying to "make my point" or force a listening from her, and simply be with her.

### Men will often focus on content, women will focus on feeling-awareness

I have gone into this personal example at some depth, but it's actually a very common situation in communication between men and women. Men will often want to focus on the *content or language of the conversation*, whereas women want an *empathic feeling response*. But it is, sadly, quite rare that either one will state their need directly – men typically for clarity, understanding, and fairness, women for empathy or feeling-awareness. Men and women often assume that their partners know what they want, and are deliberately withholding it. Everyone, fundamentally, is looking for empathy. But empathy can look different depending on a person's polarity. Empathy simply means to give a person a response that makes them feel heard and understood – but this response may be different depending on their polarity.

My advice is to learn Withholds and NVC, learn them well, and then use them to initiate a negotiation whenever you are having an emotional reaction to your partner. Be aware, however, that not everybody wants to invest that amount of time or energy in communication, or has the emotional maturity to do it. In such cases, you will need to try something different. Or just let it go.

# 38 Hexes

To **hex** someone is to challenge them, usually humorously, on an upset they are having or a belief they appear to hold. It is a lot like a "tease", but with a loving intention. The intention is often to point out to someone how they are making themselves wrong or depreciating themselves, but in a way that makes them laugh at themselves, or become more self-aware.

Their upset can be big or small. It can also be your upset that you are hexing – you can hex yourself.

Here is an example of a small hex: Your partner made a meal for you and she burned it. She offers to make another meal for you the next day. You hex her by saying, *"Are you sure it's safe for you to cook?"* Your loving intention is to defuse the fact that she burned the food, maybe to help her let go of any guilt she feels, or self-esteem issue of her cooking ability. This hex follows a typical pattern: You are **finding her right** by accepting the fact that she burnt your dinner and letting it go, where she might still feel badly about it.

Or maybe you have been asking her to do some sexual thing for a long time and she has resisted. She finally offers. You might say to her: *"Are you sure you are up for this? Can you handle it?"* This is a similar idea: You are, on the one hand, letting go of your resentment that it has taken her so long by making a joke about it, and on the other hand, lovingly challenging her to re-examine what her difficulty was.

It is possible that a hex will *"take her down"* – meaning, make her feel worse momentarily or incite a negative reaction. If that is the case, accept her reaction and let her be with it. It may be that your hex was just bad, like a bad joke. Maybe you were trying to make fun of a situation or clear an upset but you are actually putting her down. Her response to the hex will determine whether it's a good or bad hex. In the event the hex *"lands badly"* (she doesn't respond well) just apologize. It may help to process the incident with her via Withholds. A bad hex might open a healing conversation.

# 39 Anti-negotiations [Alison Armstrong]

A technique from Alison Armstrong's book, **QUEEN'S CODE**, turns the traditional notion of "negotiation" on its head, and is a helpful way to approach any kind of needs conflict inside an intimate partnership. This also is a very powerful idea.

You approach a traditional negotiation with the goal of getting the most you can while giving the least you can. Instead of this, approach a negotiation with your partner *in the spirit of giving the most you can and getting back the least you can, while still "staying within your value system" – i.e. remaining happy with the outcome, because you are coming from a place of generosity.*

If you can learn how to express a need clearly, without making her wrong and without it coming across as a demand, and provided you are open to honest feedback, it's quite possible your partner will naturally want to fulfill that need. She may also find ways of satisfying that need that are better than what you had in mind. The practices of NVC can also be helpful for this purpose.

Many sexual differences, in particular, can be resolved through the "anti-negotiation" approach. If you are generous with your woman, and she really feels your commitment to her, your attention on her and your desire to please her, she will likely reciprocate. Always "within her value system," of course, but sometimes value systems can stretch.

# 40 You don't need to get what you want if you can express what you want

The idea that *"you don't need to get what you want if you can express what you want"* comes from psychologist and Jungian analyst Strephon Kaplan Williams[12].

It is a profound truth in human relations, because **neither you nor your partner can ever fully know your desire until it has left your lips.** Human beings can only fully know themselves in relation to each other. This is why asking for what you want, or think you want, is the most important thing that you will ever do with your partner, regardless of your polarity.

Once you have asked for it, sit back and bask in the ecstasy of having spoken a deep truth about yourself. And then consider whether you still need, or even want, that thing that you thought you wanted so desperately two minutes ago. Maybe you do, maybe it has changed (in which case, speak the new need), or maybe you just needed to say it a it is gone. Or maybe it just needs to sit for a few hours or days after yo expression, and you will get new clarity.

## Why sharing your needs is so important

The reason, of course, that sharing your needs honestly and courageously with your partner is so important, is that you are giving them an opportunity to fill that need – that is, to love you – and therefore make life more wonderful for both of you. It is always a grea act of love to share your needs and wants without the demand that yo partner fulfill them. What is more, **simply sharing a need will often complete and fully satisfy the desire**. You can then completely let it go, whether your partner is able to meet that need or not. That is the meaning of Strephon Kaplan Williams' wise words.

It can be immensely freeing to state needs in a way that does not com

---

12 See THE JUNGIAN-SENOI DREAMWORK MANUAL: A STEP-BY-STEP INTRODUCTION TO WORKING WITH DREAMS by Strephon Kaplan-Williams.

across as a demand or a criticism. If your partner and you can agree to state your feelings and needs in the spirit of *"you don't need to get what you want if you can express what you want,"* it might free you both to express your needs more easily and fluently. It will defuse the fear that an expression of needs might be taken as a demand. This will help you both.

It can be valuable early on in a relationship to make a kind of **truth pact** with your partner. Ask her to be as truthful as she can with you all the time, to never be afraid of hurting your feelings, and ask her if she would be willing to receive the same from you. And explain to her also the fluidity of needs, the concept of *"you don't have to get what you want if you can express what you want,"* and that it's very important to you to have open communication in this zone.

# 41 Training Organizations

Below I list some recommended organizations which provide workshops and models that will accelerate your learning as you navigate the rocky shoals of relating to the opposite sex – and of loving anyone, for that matter. I have experienced all of these, except for Alison Armstrong's programs, which I recommend due to the brilliance of her publications.

## Shalom Mountain Retreat Center

The Shalom Mountain Retreat Center is located in the Catskills area of New York State, about two hours northwest of New York City. The center was founded by Jerry Jud in 1976 and has been running ever since. "Shalom" means "peace" in Hebrew, but the center is not otherwise connected to Judaism.

Shalom Mountain offers a variety of retreats and gatherings dedicated to calling people to become more fully alive through the creation of intentional loving community. Their core program, called a **Shalom Retreat,** runs monthly and is a 3-1/2 day residential weekend that includes elements of group process, community-building, self-expression, and celebration. These retreats are extraordinarily powerful and quite affordable. Generous scholarship are offered to those in need. They also offer programs for men, women, couples, young adults, LGBT, elders, and more. There are Shalom Mountain communities in about a dozen US cities and Canada. Check their website ShalomMountain.com.

## Non-Violent Communication (NVC)

There are courses and communities that practice NVC in many American cities, and internationally. More information is available at the Center for Non-Violent Communication website, cnvc.org

## Alison Armstrong and PAX Programs

Alison Armstrong has been researching man/woman issues and leading workshops for 20 years. Her main workshop is the QUEEN'S CODE

WORKSHOP, and she also has program for men. These programs are offered all over the United States. Check the website understandingmen. com

## Network for a New Culture (NFNC)

Network For a New Culture (NFNC) is a North American group that was originally inspired by the German intentional community ZEGG (which was, in turn, inspired by Dieter Duhm's work).

NFNC seeks to build a sustainable, violence-free culture through exploring intimacy, personal growth, transparency, radical honesty, equality, compassion, sexual freedom, and the power of community. There are currently "New Culture" centers in Washington DC, Philadelphia, Ashland Oregon, and Hawaii. Their events are absolutely wonderful, especially their "Summer camps", some of which sell out months in advance. They also offer information sessions, practice groups and community gatherings at regular intervals in all the places above. Check out the website for details: nfnc.org

## Tamera Healing Biotope (Portugal)

Tamera is an intentional community of about 170 people in Portugal. It was co-founded in 1995 by Dieter Duhm, and is hence related both to the ZEGG community in East Germany, and to the US-based Network for a New Culture (see above).

Tamera opens to visitors and students in the summer and runs programs ranging from work-study (starting at 20 € per day), month-long intensives on community-building based on the ZEGG Forum process, to their "Love School" that teaches Dieter Duhm's "free love" model, and more. Many people return every spring and stay the whole season.

## One Taste (Nicole Daedone)

One Taste was founded on the principle of Orgasmic Meditation (a variation of the Do-Date), a practice designed to get people connected to their bodies and in community. One Taste has centers in about a dozen cities in the US and internationally, and runs classes and workshop on man/woman communication and sexuality. For an introduction to this work, attend one of their fun "TurnOn" events, which you can find on their website and on Meetup.com. See the website OneTaste.us.

## Lafayette Morehouse

The Lafayette Morehouse is an intentional community in Lafayette, California. It was founded by Victor Baranco in 1968 and is still active.

Victor Baranco, who died in 2002, was an early pioneer in human sexuality and man/woman relationships. He popularized the **Do-Date**, originated many of the sexual polarity concepts and emotional communication practices discussed in this book, and inspired an entire generation of sexual educators.

The Lafayette Morehouse offers courses on sensuality, man/woman relationships, and community-building on their campus at Lafayette, California (near Oakland). There are associated groups in Atlanta, New York, and Philadelphia.

There are also related, low-cost events called **Mark Groups** in each of these cities. A Mark Group is an evening of social communication games designed for meeting people and having fun. They are great places to meet people who might be aligned with the ideas presented in this book. If you live in Asheville NC, there are similar groups called **Being Socials** (BeingSocials.com).

For more information, see the Lafayette Morehouse website (lafmore. com) or else Google my article **LAFAYETTE MOREHOUSE HISTORY**.

## Rebekah Beneteau and "Being Socials"

Rebekah Beneteau (my ex-wife) trained at the Lafayette Morehouse, and also has extensive training at Shalom Mountain in the Skills and Principle of Loving. She approaches personal development and self-actualization through the power of pleasure and of discovering and expressing your authentic sexual nature. She runs workshops and programs in Asheville, NC and other places. She also runs the Asheville Being Socials groups, which are similar to the Hot Seats Game. Find her at pleasureevolution.com

## Mama Gena

Mama Gena was trained by Victor Baranco. Her classic book **MAMA GENA'S SCHOOL OF WOMANLY ARTS: USING THE POWER OF PLEASURE**

TO HAVE YOUR WAY WITH THE WORLD teaches women fundamental attitudes and practices for identifying their desire, having fun no matter what, making pleasure goals important, playing with masculine resistance, and much more. It is a great book for a woman who understands the power of pleasure and wants to leverage that inherent feminine strength into deeper relationships with men and greater happiness and success all around.

Mama Gena also runs live retreats for women. Check out her website mamagenas.com

# 42 Bibliography

### Alison Armstrong

Alison Armstrong's QUEEN'S CODE lays down the fundamental attitude beliefs and communication practices that feminine people can use to b successful in relationship with a man within the sexual polarity model presented in this book. Alison has several other books as well. Look fo them on Amazon.

### Steve & Vera Bodansky

Steve and Vera were trained by Victor Baranco. They have one of the finest books on the philosophy of man/woman, including the approac healthy attitudes, acknowledgment of your partner, marriage and fam within a sexually polarized relationship, sexual techniques, and more. The book is called TO BED OR NOT TO BED: WHAT MEN WANT, WHAT WOMEN WANT, HOW GREAT SEX HAPPENS. If you have enjoyed my book I would recommend the Bodansky's book as the next stage of your research.

Steve and Vera also have several books covering advanced sexual techniques, notably EXTENDED MASSIVE ORGASM: HOW YOU CAN GIVE AND RECEIVE INTENSE SEXUAL PLEASURE. I recommend it to guide the next steps of your sexual exploration.

### David Deida

David Deida is a brilliant Tantra master and sexual educator. His class book THE WAY OF THE SUPERIOR MAN: A SPIRITUAL GUIDE TO MASTERI THE CHALLENGES OF WOMEN, WORK, AND SEXUAL DESIRE has inspired thousands of men to greater honesty, authenticity and integrity with their partners. He also has books for women including DEAR LOVER: A WOMAN'S GUIDE TO MEN, SEX, AND LOVE'S DEEPEST BLISS.

Deida has many other books, but start with those two. An interesting narrative on the education of a Tantra master is found in his autobiography **WILD NIGHTS**. Other personal stories are found in **THE ENLIGHTENED SEX MANUAL: SEXUAL SKILLS FOR THE SUPERIOR LOVER**.

### Marshall Rosenberg

Marshall Rosenberg is the author of **NONVIOLENT COMMUNICATION: A LANGUAGE OF LIFE** which is the basic textbook for Non-Violent Communication. Reading the book is excellent, but finding a teacher, practice group or weekend workshop is even better. NVC training is offered in over 60 countries and is usually extremely affordable.

### Dieter Duhm

Duhm is a brilliant writer, philosopher and social activist, and the founder of the **Tamera** Healing Biotope in Portugal. His book **THE SACRED MATRIX** lays out in a very compelling way a path to planetary healing that includes new models of human loving and sexuality. **EROS UNREDEEMED** is a magnificent analysis of our cultural oppression around sexuality, and the possibility of creating a new model of love and sexuality. The community **Tamera**, which he co-founded in 1995, offers many courses and internships and is quite affordable. Duhm is a personal mentor and great inspiration of mine.

### Patricia Taylor

In addition to Steve & Vera Bodansky's books, see Patricia Taylor's **EXPANDED ORGASM: SOAR TO ECSTASY AT YOUR LOVER'S EVERY TOUCH**. Patti Taylor is Morehouse-trained and runs workshops in San Francisco, New York City and elsewhere.

### Nicole Daedone

(See also the OneTaste entry in the previous chapter). Nicole has several books, including **SLOW SEX: THE ART AND CRAFT OF THE FEMALE ORGASM** and **HOW TO OM: A STEP BY STEP GUIDE TO ORGASMIC MEDITATION**. Nicole Daedone was also trained by Victor Baranco and her **Orgasmic Meditation** is a variation of the do-date technique. Google her fun Ted talk.

### Mark Manson

Manson's **MODELS** is the best men's dating and seduction book. See Chapter 11.

## A final bombshell: Tantric Sex and Non-Ejaculatory Orgasm

I would encourage you to research the practice of *Non-Ejaculatory Orgasm* – and especially if you are a man older than 40. This type orgasm does not involve the release of sperm and is one of the fundamental Tantric practices. It is accomplished through breathing, visualization, and energy-circulation techniques with your partner. See David Deida's **WAY OF THE SUPERIOR MAN** and **THE ENLIGHTENED SEX MANUAL**. Also look for books and lectures by Mantak Chia and Margot Anand.

# Acknowledgements

Many people have made this book possible:

All my teachers and mentors discussed in these pages. I walk in the footsteps of giants. I hope they would be pleased with me.

My intimate partners, especially Rebekah and Zahra: you have taught me everything I know. No words can express my gratitude.

My wonderful family and friends who continue to love me, even when they do not always understand me. This is the definition of love.

John, Robert, Nancy and Philippa: human angels whom I try to emulate,

If you have enjoyed this book, please visit our website and community at AsLoversDo.com. You will find there support for creating your own As LOVERS DO book club.

On the website you also find video instructions for running your own community-building and networking events based on a process called Hot Seats. The Hot Seats game is a social conversation game designed for meeting people and having fun, which will expand your community and help you create a lifestyle aligned with the ideas in this book.

Made in the USA
Las Vegas, NV
24 April 2023

71052911R00118